CONDOMS

Edited by

ADRIAN MINDEL

*Professor of Sexual Health Medicine, University of
Sydney and New South Wales, Sydney Hospital,
Sydney, Australia*

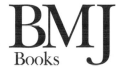

First published in 2000

BMJ Books is an imprint of the BMJ Publishing Group,
BMA House, Tavistock Square, London WC1H 9JR

www.bmjbooks.com

British Library Cataloguing in Publication Data

A catalogue record for this book is available from the British Library

ISBN 0-7279-1267-4

Typeset by J&L Composition Ltd, Filey, North Yorkshire
Printed and bound by J W Arrowsmith Ltd, Bristol

Contents

Contributors

R J Aitken
Professor, Department of Biological Sciences, University of Newcastle, Callaghan, New South Wales, 2308 Australia.

Gina Dallabetta
Director, Technical Support, HIV/AIDS Prevention and Care Department, Family Health International, Arlington, VA, USA.

Claudia Estcourt
Senior Lecturer, Academic Unit of Sexual Health Medicine, Universities of Sydney and New South Wales, Sydney Hospital, Sydney, Australia.

Gaston Farr
Associate Director, Clinical Trials Division, Family Health International, Research Triangle Park, NC, USA.

Madaline P Feinberg
Technical Support Group, HIV/AIDS Prevention and Care Department, Family Health International, Arlington, VA, USA.

John Gerofi
Managing Director, Enersol Consulting Engineers, Annandale, New South Wales, Australia.

Anne Grunseit
Researcher, National Centre in HIV Social Research, The University of New South Wales, Sydney, Australia.

Philip Harvey
President, DKT International, Washington, DC, USA.

D J Jeffries
Professor of Virology, Department of Medical Microbiology, St Bartholomew's and Royal London School of Medicine and Dentistry, London, UK.

Anne M Johnson
Professor of Epidemiology, Department of Sexually Transmitted Diseases, Royal Free and University College Medical School, London, UK.

Philip Kestelman
Freelance condomologist, former Europe Regional Medical Secretary, International Planned Parenthood Federation, London, UK.

Susan Kippax
Professor and Director, National Centre in HIV Social Research, The University of New South Wales, Sydney, Australia.

Milton Lewis
NHMRC Senior Research Fellow, Department of Public Health and Community Medicine, University of Sydney, Australia.

Adrian Mindel
Professor of Sexual Health Medicine, Universities of Sydney and New South Wales, Sydney Hospital, Sydney, Australia.

Juliet Richters
Research Fellow, National Centre in HIV Social Research, The University of New South Wales, Sydney, Australia.

William Schellstede
Senior Vice President, Family Health International, Arlington, VA, USA.

Brenda Spencer
Unit for the Evaluation of Prevention Programmes, University Institute of Social and Preventative Medicine, Lausanne, Switzerland.

James Trussell
Professor of Economics and Public Affairs, Princeton University, Princeton, NJ, USA.

Anne M Young
Programme Associate, Management Sciences for Health, Boston, MA, USA.

Preface

Sexual intercourse is an enjoyable and fulfilling activity for most adults. However, unwanted pregnancies or the acquisition of sexually transmitted infections (STIs) constitute an important risk to the personal happiness and well-being of some individuals and a significant risk to public health. The World Health Organization (WHO) has estimated that worldwide over 12 million adults a year are infected with syphilis, over 60 million with gonorrhoea, and over 80 million with chlamydia. In addition the WHO calculated that there were over 30 million individuals living with HIV/AIDS at the end of 1997, with millions more becoming infected each year. These infections occur around the world; however, developing countries suffer a disproportionate burden. The burden on women and the social and financial cost to the community from unwanted or unintended pregnancies is colossal, with an estimated 50 million abortions and 30 million unintended pregnancies annually.

Condoms are a highly effective, cheap, and largely side-effect free, method of contraception. In addition, when used for every act of sexual intercourse, they offer a high degree of protection against many STIs, including HIV, gonorrhoea, and chlamydia. Condoms have become an everyday part of life in most parts of the developed world with ready availability from numerous commercial outlets, including pharmacies, super-markets, and fuel service stations. Yet in many developing, and in some developed countries, social, religious, political, and financial constraints restrict their availability; also personal likes, dislikes, and prejudices limit their use.

The aim of this book is to bring together the vast amount of diverse information about condoms into a concise and readable format, and by doing so to promote condom use and thereby decrease unwanted pregnancies and reduce the spread and consequences of STIs. The information presented ranges from the manufacture and quality standards of condoms; through to the efficacy in the prevention of pregnancy, STIs and HIV; population surveys; barriers to use; social marketing and the practical aspects of how to use a condom. Additional chapters include female condoms, plastic condoms, the history of condoms, spermicides and microbicides, and condoms for anal sex.

I believe the book will be of interest and value to a variety of health care providers, including family planning doctors and nurses, physicians concerned with sexually transmitted diseases (genitourinary medicine) and infectious diseases, public health physicians, social planners, health economists, and non-government agencies promoting family planning, sexual and reproductive health.

Multi-author books are fraught with difficulty and I am grateful to the contributors for putting up with my relentless demands for changes, and to the publishers for their willingness to wholeheartedly embrace this project. If this book results in the prevention of just one per cent of unwanted pregnancies per year or the prevention of transmission of one per cent of new cases of HIV, it will have achieved its objective.

Adrian Mindel
Sydney Hospital,
Australia

1 A brief history of condoms

MILTON LEWIS

Introduction

The role of the male condom as both contraceptive and preventive of disease was established in Europe in the eighteenth century. Since then, its image has suffered from negative associations in each area of use. Identified as a prophylactic against sexually acquired diseases in a context of illicit sex, its use as a preventive of pregnancy has suffered. Identified as a contraceptive in a context of pronatalism, its use as a preventive of infection has suffered. The fluctuating fortunes of this device in the last 250 to 300 years may be usefully viewed against the background of this double stigmatisation. "Invented" in response to the epidemic of syphilis which swept Europe from the close of the fifteenth century (and soon spread to Asia), the condom has been enjoying a revival of popularity in response to the pandemic of HIV/AIDS that has swept the world in the late twentieth century.

Origins

Penis protectors were worn in Ancient Egypt and by some preliterate tribal peoples. However, they were not used for contraception but for a variety of other purposes including protection in combat, decoration, or as indicators of status.[1,2] The Ancient Greeks used a variety of contraceptives including barrier methods, but there is no evidence of sheaths being employed.[3] The male or female condom may have been used in imperial Rome but the evidence is slim, arising from a legend about Minos, King of

1

Crete, related by Antoninus Liberalis (fl. 150 AD?). A goat's bladder was employed by a woman as a female condom into which Minos shed his serpent-bearing semen, notorious for injuring his sexual partners. He then safely impregnated his wife, Pasiphae. Himes concluded from this thin base of evidence that some form of condom was used in Rome but not widely.[1]

The ancient civilisations of East Asia may also have employed condoms from an early date. Men in China sometimes employed a cover for the glans. This was intended to be a preventive of conception rather than a protection against infection.[4] The Japanese, traditionally, employed a hard condom, a "kabuto-gata or helmet [for the glans] made of tortoise shell or horn which not only gives the woman much satisfaction but [it is claimed] also prevents conception at the same time".[1] The Dutch, who were trading with the Japanese from the seventeenth century, are thought to have introduced to Japan a new type of condom: " . . . a Kyotai is made of thin leather, and foreigners call it Ryurusakku [perhaps from the Dutch, roede-zak]".[1]

The epidemic of syphilis, which spread across Europe from the end of the fifteenth century, gave rise to the first published account of the condom. In De Morbo Gallico (1564), Fallopius (1523–62) described a sheath of linen he claimed to have invented to protect men against syphilis: "As often as a man has intercourse, he should use a small linen cloth made to fit the glans, and draw forward the prepuce over the glans".[5] The medical writer, Hercules Saxonia, described in 1597 a sheath made of linen which was soaked in a solution and then allowed to dry before use.[6,7]

Himes claimed that in 1671, Mme de Sévigné (1626–96), in a letter to her daughter, mentioned a sheath made of gold-beaters skin.[1] But a contemporary scholar, WE Kruck, has declared the letter never existed.[2] The use of the linen glans cover, as a contraceptive, is mentioned as early as 1655 in "L'Escole Des Filles", a manual of erotic technique.[6] The English venereologist, Daniel Turner (1667–1741) wrote in 1717, "The 'Condum' . . . [is] the best . . . preservative our Libertines have found . . . and yet, by reason of its blunting the Sensation, I have heard some of them acknowledge, that they had often chose to risque a 'Clap', rather than engage 'cum Hastis sic Clypeatis' [with spears thus sheathed]."[5] Jean Astruc (1684–1766), the French venereologist, condemned the English libertines' use of the animal membrane condom in 1736: "Surely it is far better . . . to partake the pleasures of venery with permission and safety, than to make use of so filthy and nasty an invention."[6]

The term, "condom"

The first published use of the word, "condum" was in a 1706 poem, probably composed by Lord Belhaven (1656–1708). The anonymous author of a 1708 poem referred to "matchless Condon" whose fame would "last as long as Condon is a Name".[6] The debate about the existence of Condom (or Cundum, Condum, Condon or Conton) has a long history. Condom was allegedly a physician in the time of Charles II, who invented the device to help his King prevent the birth of more illegitimate children. Modern authorities are inclined to reject the idea for lack of conclusive evidence, but Bernstein concluded that "Cundum" was more likely to have been an army officer than a physician and "popularised" the device some time between 1680 and 1717.[1,8] Others have also attempted to explain the name. Ferdy suggested condom was from the name of a village in the Department of Gers, France. He later proposed that it was derived from the Latin, "condere" (to hide, to protect). Richter believed that condom was derived from the Persian "kendü", a storage vessel made of animal intestines, and that an (anonymous) medieval scholar had wittily Latinised the name.[1] Himes dismissed both Richter's and Ferdy's explanations as far-fetched.[1]

The condom in the eighteenth century

There are abundant references to the condom in eighteenth-century literature. In "The Petticoat" (1716), Joseph Gay affirms that "The New Machine a sure defence shall prove/And guard the sex against the Harm of Love".[7] White Kennett (d. 1740) wrote in 1723 in "Armour", "Happy the Man, who in his Pocket keeps/Whether with Green or Scarlet Ribband bound/A well-made C. . . . He, nor dreads the Ills/Of Shankers or Cordee, or Buboes Dire!"[6]

Both Casanova (1725–98) and James Boswell (1740–95) commonly used condoms. Casanova appears to have employed them for contraception as well as for protection against infection.[6] In London in 1762, young Boswell picked up a girl in the Strand but since she had no condom, he abstained from intercourse and afterwards "trembled at the danger" from which he had escaped. Early

3

in 1763, he picked up a woman in St James's Park: "For the first time did I engage in armour, which I found but a dull satisfaction."[9]

In the second half of the eighteenth century, a trade in hand-made condoms flourished in London. In a handbill of 1776, Mrs Philips advertised condoms for sale at the Green Canister in Half-Moon Street, in the Strand. She offered to supply "apothecaries, chymists, druggists etc." as well as, "Ambassadors, foreigners, gentlemen and captains of ships . . . going abroad".[1] But output must have been severely limited by the nature of the manufacturing process involved, described in Dunglinson's nineteenth-century *Dictionary of Medical Science*: "The intestinal caecum of a sheep, soaked for some hours in water . . . scraped carefully to abstract the mucous membrane . . . exposed to the vapour of burning brimstone, and afterwards washed with soap and water. It is then blown up, dried, cut to the length of seven or eight inches, and bordered at the open end with a riband".[10] "Baudruches fines" were further refined by being drawn over oiled moulds after being brimstoned; "Baudruches superfines" were first perfumed and then placed on a glass mould and polished by rubbing with a glass. "Baudruches superfines doubles" were made by drawing another caecum over the original; both being moist, they adhered to each other.[6] Figure 1.1 shows early condoms.

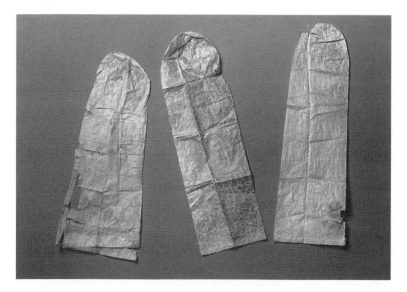

Figure 1.1   Early condoms made of a caecum of a sheep. Source: Contraception Museum, Canada.

Nineteenth-century developments

The use of condoms was affected by technological, economic and social developments in nineteenth-century Europe and the United States. While the rise of the birth control movement and the transition to lower fertility, on the one hand, and vulcanization of rubber and mass production, on the other, promoted their use, continuing stigma and probably cost (for working class people) worked against their extensive spread.

The birth control movement

The birth control movement developed most strongly in Britain from where it spread to the United States and Continental Europe. Thomas Malthus' (1766–1834) ideas about the need to restrain population growth were taken up by reformers like Francis Place, Richard Carlile, Robert Dale Owen, and George and Charles Drysdale. Neo-Malthusians advocated birth control as the way to solve the problem of poverty. In 1826, a publication by Carlile (1790–1843), the first book in England on birth control, discussed withdrawal, the sponge for women, and the "baudruche" for men.[5] American, Charles Knowlton (1800–50) discussed condoms but did not endorse their use as contraceptives, seeing them as primarily for prevention of syphilis[11]; while Charles Drysdale (1829–1907) found them not only disgusting but reductive of pleasure. The sponge was the generally preferred Neo-Malthusian contraceptive, although in the latter decades of the nineteenth century the diaphragm and soluble pessary became available. The vulcanisation of rubber made available comparatively cheap, rubber condoms.[3]

Condoms played a part in the fertility decline in Europe and also in European settlements overseas – the United States and Australia – in the last decades of the nineteenth and first decades of the twentieth century, but how large a part is uncertain. In the extensive literature on the relationship between social and economic factors and the nineteenth-century fertility decline, different factors have been stressed by different researchers: change to marriages based on mutual affection; a rising living standard and the wish to promote that by limiting families; decline in the influence of religion with its opposition to family limitation; education of women; reduction in child mortality with less need for large families; feminism and the role of women; and birth control. Certainly, the speed of the decline suggests that some form of birth control was being used on a wide scale, but to what extent this involved new access to contraceptive knowledge or new motivation to use already known methods is uncertain.[12]

The Australian fertility decline as a case study

Crude birth rates in Australia declined from 43.3 per 1000 in 1862 to 35 in 1877, and to 27.3 in 1900. The marked decline has been attributed to a variety of changes of shorter or longer duration. First, the introduction of compulsory schooling in the 1870s reduced the value of children as labour. Second, the major economic depression of the 1890s reduced incomes for many. Third, lower child mortality may have induced parents to reduce the births required to reach the desired number of offspring. Fourth, longer-term change in the status of women – "domestic feminism" – probably gave them more influence in issues concerning children. Finally, the diffusion of information about birth control, and some new techniques, impacted upon fertility.[12] Certainly, the New South Wales Royal Commission on the Decline of the Birth-Rate, 1903–4, which attracted considerable national and even international attention, heard evidence suggesting the main methods by which fertility was reduced in the previous two decades were widespread practice of withdrawal, considerable resort to abortion, and the use of douches, sponges, and soluble pessaries, with some use of rubber condoms.[13,14] The Commission heard that members of every social class practised birth control but it was more common among the middle and upper classes. This was in part due to the cost of the manufactured contraceptives. "Lambert's Paragon Sheath", the "Pessary Capote" and the "Mensinga Check Pessary" (diaphragm) cost respectively seven shillings and six pence, eight shillings and six pence, and five shillings. Such outlays must have been difficult for lower middle class wage earners whose total weekly income was two to three pounds, let alone for working class men.[13]

Seven brands of condoms were marketed in New South Wales around the turn of the century: "Malthus Sheaths" (six shillings and six pence per dozen); "Transparent Skin Sheaths" (eight shillings and six pence per dozen); "Durrant's French Letters"; "Grecian Caps" (worn over the glans; three shillings and six pence each); "Lambert's Paragon Sheaths"; "Lambert's Combined Pessary and Sheath"; and "Never Rips". They do not seem to have been greatly popular as contraceptives. Robert Scot-Skirving, a leading Sydney doctor, told the Royal Commission that condoms were the third most popular method. They seem to have been used as venereal disease preventives as much as contraceptives.[13,15] Moreover, large numbers do not appear to have been sold. H.S. Levy of the wholesale druggists, Elliott Brothers, Sydney told the Royal Commission that pharmacists in Sydney (population of 482 000 in 1901) and all country towns stocked condoms. But his firm sold to retail chemists the comparatively small number of 150 gross a year which, he believed, was about half of all condoms sold in New South Wales. A number of Sydney retail pharmacists told the Commission that condoms were used more for disease prevention than contraception; and some stocked "French letters with things on top" ("ticklers") but few were sold.[15]

The growth of the condom industry

The American, Charles Goodyear's discovery of vulcanization in 1839 permitted the mass production of rubber condoms. In Britain, E Lambert and Sons of Dalston became the main producer in the later nineteenth century, being established in 1877, the same year as the Malthusian League, the first birth control

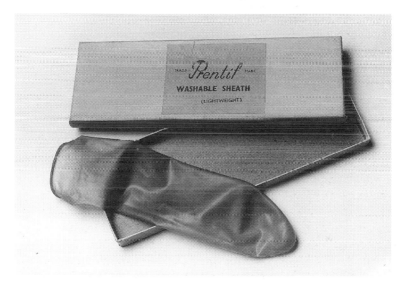

Figure 1.2 Early rubber condom, advertised as re-usable.
Source: Contraception Museum, Canada.

body in the world, was founded.[16] Until the 1920s, most condoms were manufactured by hand-dipping from rubber cement. They were not only of dubious quality but aged quickly. In Akron, Ohio, in 1919, Frederick Killian initiated hand-dipping from natural rubber latex. Latex condoms had the market advantage of a life of three to five years before ageing; also they were odourless and usually less thick than the crepe rubber products. The new condoms enjoyed great expansion of sales. By the mid-1930s, the fifteen largest makers in the United States were producing 1.5 million a day. After the first world war, German output also grew dramatically, one firm alone marketing 24 million annually. Mass marketing was assisted there (and in Holland) by sale through coin vending machines; and when the machines were introduced in the United States, druggists began to lose ground to other outlets.[1,17]

Growth of the market was promoted by the virtual nullification of the nineteenth-century Federal Comstock Acts which had made illegal interstate trade in condoms. When in the late 1920s Merrill Youngs sued Lee and Company of Chicago for trademark misuse, the United States Court of Appeals for the Second Circuit ruled that where not contrary to local law, contraception was a legitimate medical activity, and sale of condoms through drug outlets was legal.[17]

An Australian company, Ansell, was eventually to become an important supplier of the international market. The Dunlop Pneumatic Tyre Company of Melbourne made tyres, hoses, proofed clothing, and condoms. But in 1905, Nicholas Fitzgerald, company chairman and Papal knight, decided to cease producing condoms. Eric Ansell, an employee, purchased the condom plant and began production. After trials in 1929, he was the first in Australia to import liquid latex. In 1969, Dunlop Australia (later Pacific Dunlop) acquired Ansell and the company became Ansell International in 1977. In the American market, the value of Ansell condom sales grew from $4.6 million in 1982 to $19.4 million in 1988. The latter figure should be viewed against the following market shares for 1988: Carter-Wallace, $109.8 million; Schmid Laboratories, $73.1 million; and others, $43.7 million. In 1989, with most of its condom output being produced in its American factories, Ansell International ceased production in Australia. Ansell was then supplying three million gross of condoms per year to the United States Agency for International Development, most of the condoms purchased by this aid agency to assist birth control policies in developing countries.[17,18]

Changing use of the condom

Greater use of condoms in the twentieth century was not just a result of technological development and of economic factors like mass marketing and lower prices. It was part of a spiralling relationship between contraception and a revolution in nonmarital sexual behaviour: contraceptives encouraged sexual activity and the new acceptability of sexual freedom encouraged contraception. There is evidence of a significant growth of nonmarital sex by women in the early twentieth century in the United States. Alfred Kinsey found that the percentage of women having premarital intercourse was double for those born in 1900–29 compared with those born before 1900. The experience of troops in the first world war also had a large impact on condom use in the United States and elsewhere. Unimpressed by the British and French military's focus on treatment, the American Expeditionary Force took up the New Zealand forces' policy of prevention of venereal disease through frequent inspections and early treatment, and provision of chemical prophylaxis and condoms. Military service in the first world war promoted knowledge of condoms, not only as a source of disease prevention but also as contraceptives. The civilian market in the United States for condoms expanded in the immediate postwar years. A study in Baltimore found where before the war, two to three million were sold annually, about 6.25 million were sold in the mid-1920s; and perhaps 50 per cent of purchasers were unmarried.[19,20]

The norm of the small family was firmly established in the interwar period. The cohort of American women who married in the 1920s had fewer offspring than any in the period from the 1880s to the 1950s. The crude birth rate in Britain, which had been 34.1 per 1000 in 1870–2 and 24.5 in 1910–12, fell to 15.8 in 1930–2. Middle class, English couples using contraceptive appliances increased between 1910 and 1930 from 9 to 40 per cent, and working class from 1 to 28 per cent. In order of popularity the methods used in the 1930s were withdrawal, sheath, safe period, and pessaries.[3] But the condom still carried a double stigma: on the one hand, its use as a contraceptive by respectable couples was handicapped by association with "illicit" sex; and on the other, its use as a VD preventive was handicapped by medical and official deference to pronatalist opinion. In the United States in the 1930s, at a time of great economic hardship, Thomas Parran, head of the Federal Public Health Service, and other important officials would not speak publicly in support of birth control. Parran saw VD as the most important public health problem of the time, yet he was silent about the use of condoms as prophylactics. The American Social Hygiene Association (ASHA) took a moralistic approach to VD control, as did the National Council for Combating Venereal Diseases (NCCVD) in Britain. ASHA set its face against personal prophylaxis.[19,21,22] In Britain, the same reticence about personal prophylaxis (including condoms) was prevalent. Even the Royal Commission on Venereal Diseases, 1913–16, which proposed an enlightened approach to VD control, failed to discuss personal prophylaxis in its final report. In the interwar years, the NCCVD carried on a public battle with the Society for the Prevention of Venereal Disease, which vigorously advocated personal prophylaxis.[22,23]

Official concern about the effect of VD on military efficiency promoted the use of condoms during the second world war. In occupied France, the Germans required condoms to be used in brothels; and condoms were issued to Australian troops.[20] The British Government did not become active in VD control until, with large numbers of American troops arriving in 1942, the incidence of VD increased significantly. British condoms were not popular with the Americans who considered them too small.[20] The American military authorities quickly adopted personal prophylaxis through condoms and chemical treatments, although this drew much fire from Catholic and other moralistic critics. In fact, premarital sexual relations in all three countries were becoming more common as part of a long-term trend, and this trend was reinforced by war-time conditions of enhanced risk of death and greater social independence for women.[19,21]

In the second half of the twentieth century, the condom has enjoyed mixed fortunes as disease preventive and contraceptive. Data are available on condom use by married couples in Australia, 1935–71. As the main method of family planning, condoms were employed by 21 per cent of all users in 1935–9 but only 9 per cent in 1970–1, with the decline accelerating in the 1960s as use of the pill and IUDs increased. When Australia is compared with Britain and the United States, it is clear that the condom was more commonly used in the latter two countries. In Australia, as the main method for married couples, condoms were employed by 17 per cent of all users in 1955–9. In Britain in 1959–60, they were used by 52 per cent of couples. In the United States (as the most recent method), they were employed by 27 per cent in 1955 and 18 per cent in 1965. An important reason for the greater use of condoms in Britain than Australia was that the marketing of condoms, except by pharmacists, was illegal in Australia from the late 1930s, whereas in Britain condoms were also sold by barbers and surgical appliance stores.[14]

In 1986 a national survey of Australian women, 20–59 years of age, was carried out to determine contraceptive methods (Table 1.1). It revealed that condom use was low, overall, although use among older women was higher:[24]

Quality of condoms

The United States Food, Drug and Cosmetics Act, 1938 provided for regulation of medical devices, but it was only in the 1976 amendments to the Act that condoms came under regulation. Even then, regulation was not strictly enforced because condom use was not growing significantly, and the results of defects were not seen as catastrophic. With the appearance of HIV/AIDS, however, the situation changed dramatically and from 1986 condom standards were more stringently enforced.[17] In 1964, Britain had introduced a standard for condoms. In the same year Canberra Consumers Incorporated carried out a survey of brands commonly available in Australia and found that they had failure rates of up to 29 per cent while the then British standard allowed one per cent. When a more stringent British

Table 1.1   National survey of Australian women in 1986 showing distribution of contraceptive methods (per cent) in ever used and ever-users only used categories

Method	Ever	Ever-users only[a]
Pill	72	61
IUD	16	11
Spermicides	4	(17)
Condom	10	17
Diaphragm	9	22
Rhythm	6	(38)
Withdrawl	4	(57)

[a] Values in brackets indicate fewer than 50 ever-users.
Source: Santow (1991).[24]

standard, requiring a maximum failure rate of 0.5 per cent, was introduced in 1972, an Australian draft standard identical to it was put in place. In 1973, a survey of commonly used brands was carried out in Sydney. Apart from one batch, which was so deteriorated the condoms could not be unrolled, the tested brands averaged 2.3 per cent "serious failures" (tears anywhere and holes anywhere except in the 3 cm nearest the rim), well above the permitted rate.[25]

A decade and a half later, with the condom a critical component of HIV/AIDS prevention, concern about quality grew. An Australian condom standard published in 1976 became mandatory in 1986, and soon afterwards the new international standard, modified here to render it stricter, was adopted. In a new study, 28 condom lines were tested, of which 6 initially failed the inflation test but 3 of these lines passed after 200 more condoms had been tested. The 28 lines performed, overall, better than the condoms tested in 1973: out of the 28 lines, 2 did not pass the test for leakage but all met the standards for length and for width.[26,27]

Condoms and the advent of HIV/AIDS

From the early 1960s, use of condoms as a contraceptive device declined as the hormonal pill, the IUD and sterilisation became more popular. The availability of antibiotic cures for major sexually transmitted infections and medical preference for case-finding and treatment rather than personal prevention discouraged their use as preventives of infection. Moreover, the emphasis on spontaneity in sex in the "sexual revolution" was antipathetic to condom use. The survival of long-standing moralistic judgments that condoms encouraged "illicit" sex, and media unwillingness to advertise condoms, also worked against their use.[28] But with the coming of HIV/AIDS as a pandemic disease, the condom became central to prevention by means of safer sex practices. The humble condom enjoyed a renaissance of global proportions.

The advent of the pandemic led to reassessment of law and policy relating to condoms. In Australia, the National HIV/AIDS Strategy stated " . . . it is essential that they are available in a wide range of settings . . . The legal standards applicable to condoms will be reviewed in the light of their use as a barrier to HIV."[27] AIDS affected marketing in Britain. The London International Group, which was the maker of Durex and the major producer of condoms purchased in Britain, was reported to be, in the mid-1980s, unwilling to target the gay market for fear of the effect on its image. Into the breach stepped Mates, a condom brand marketed from 1987 as a non-profit-making, cheaper competitor for Durex. Mates condoms were sold to family planning clinics and large numbers were given to HIV/AIDS organisations for free distribution. More than 20 per cent of the market was captured after only one year. While other makers largely ignored gays, Mates promoted condom use in gay newspapers, as well as women's magazines, and thereby did a great deal publicly to promote safer sex practices. Moreover, Mates persuaded women to purchase condoms, an unprecedented market breakthrough.[16] But the London Rubber Company has continued to dominate the condom market in the 1990s, having an 83 per cent share by value.[29] The retail market was worth 53 million pounds in 1994. London International recently introduced Avanti, the stronger polyurethane condom for men. At eight dollars for a pack of six in the United States (the latex condom cost three dollars) Avanti did well to win a three per cent market share in a short time.[30]

In Britain, the condom became more popular as a contraceptive because of HIV/AIDS. By the early 1990s, 25.9 per cent of women and 36.9 per cent of men were reporting use of the condom in the previous year. More strikingly, from 1985 to 1991 there was a marked increase in the proportions of men and women reporting use of condoms at first intercourse.[31]

In the 1980s, Japan was using about 25 per cent of the world's condoms. This is not surprising, given the fact that oral contraceptives were not legal, voluntary sterilisation was restricted and Japanese women were not happy with methods entailing touching of their own genitals. Japan was not only a country of high condom use (51 per cent using, 1979) like Britain (18 per cent, 1976) but it was early acquainted with the modern condom. Rubber condoms were introduced to Japan soon after the Meiji restoration in 1868 exposed the country to the modern world. A Japanese tradition lending itself to widespread condom marketing was the visiting salesman who would leave a box of medicines for household use. The Family Planning Association, established in 1955, distributed love boxes containing condoms (for which payment was left in the box).[1,32] By 1987, almost 77 per cent of couples in the reproductive age-group were using condoms.[33]

In response to the AIDS pandemic, WHO sought to promote condoms as the principal preventive method for those practising high-risk sex behaviours. In Asia, countries like Bangladesh, China, India, Hong Kong, Singapore, and Taiwan had achieved by the beginning of the 1990s acceptance of condoms among sizeable proportions of the reproductive age population. But the great challenge in other countries of the region lay in overcoming the negative associations. India had initiated promotional campaigns for target groups. However, in Indonesia, promotion in the 1980s had only raised use from 0.83 per cent in 1980 to 1.65 per cent in 1984. The condom's association with promiscuity, taboos on discussion of sexuality, and male dominance in family matters all worked against greater use. Prostitutes and brothel owners saw condom use as an unattainable goal because of strong client resistance and intense competition within the industry.[33,34] In Sri Lanka, on the other hand, promotion of male condoms was well established thanks to a family planning programme heritage. In Thailand, while contraceptive use was low, use as a disease preventive was high. Hong Kong had a high level of condom use for contraceptive purposes, but efforts were being made to reach tourists as part of AIDS prevention work.[33]

Pacific Island nations like Fiji, Vanuatu, and the Solomon Islands faced cultural and economic barriers to increased condom use. In Fiji, user and government financial constraints were the primary impediment. In Vanuatu, health posts distributed condoms for contraception but only to married persons. The Solomons had a pronatalist culture.[33] In Africa, developing countries were supplied by international health bodies and USAID, and supplies increased dramatically between 1987 and 1990: WHO from 0 to 62 million; International Planned Parenthood Federation, from 1.8 to 6.5 million; UN Population Fund from 10.2 to 20.5 million; and USAID from 33.8 to 175.5 million.[35]

Surveys in Britain and Australia in the 1980s and 90s showed contraceptive condom use decreased with increasing age.[31,36] But despite the impact of HIV/AIDS publicity and education, some young people were clearly refusing to use condoms for disease protection. The authors of an Australian survey of attitudes of teenagers and young adults in the late 1980s proposed that to be effective, health educators had to offer young women role models who made sex conditional on the use of condoms.[36] An authority on Australian sexual health in the 1990s pointed out that while the youth generally seemed well informed about HIV/AIDS, teenage boys were more able than girls to assert their sexual needs; in

14

raising the issue of condom use, young girls found they risked being labelled as "sluts".[37]

HIV/AIDS has progressed more slowly among female sex workers in developed than in developing countries. Condom use has been central to containment of the epidemic among sex workers. In a 1985 survey of female sex workers attending the Sydney STD Centre, the largest sexual health clinic in Australia, only 11 per cent used condoms with clients and nonpaying partners. Centre staff believed that fewer than 5 per cent of women in the trade insisted that clients use condoms. By 1987, AIDS information campaigns and educational work had produced a dramatic increase in condom use by parlour prostitutes (female and male). A 1988 survey found 88 per cent of female prostitutes in New South Wales were using condoms with all clients and 32.7 per cent for all heterosexual contacts. An early 1990s study of female sex workers found 98 per cent always used condoms with clients.[38,39]

HIV/AIDS also focussed attention on condom availability. A clear barrier to greater use is a narrow range of sales outlets. Whereas in the United States and Britain, condoms could be purchased from a wide range of outlets, in some Australian States in the early 1990s legislation still restricted distribution. There were no restrictions on widespread distribution in Victoria, South Australia, Western Australia, the Northern Territory, and the Australian Capital Territory (ACT). But in New South Wales (NSW), while condoms might be sold from vending machines, such machines could not be located in or near a church, a school, or a residence. In Queensland, while vending machines were allowed from 1988, supply was still prohibited in all schools and Technical and Further Education colleges.[27]

The availability of condoms in prisons was another contentious issue, but by the later 1990s there had been some progress. Condoms are now available in all men's correctional institutions in NSW. They are not available in Queensland, Northern Territory, Tasmanian, or South Australian prisons. In Victoria, machines dispensing condoms are located in prisons where residential, visiting facilities are provided for prisoners and their families. In the ACT, inmates are offered condoms on entry into the correctional facility. A trial has begun in two Western Australian prisons, whereby condoms and lubricants are sold to all prisoners over the age of 21 years (personal communication from M. Argy, Government lawyer, Human Rights branch, Attorney General's Department, Canberra, 7 May 1998).

An important development in the 1990s was the marketing of the polyurethane female condom. Stronger than the latex male condom, used properly, it is very effective in prevention of pregnancy and as a barrier to STIs, including HIV. Empowering of women, it is widely perceived as a significant tool in prevention of HIV/AIDS especially in poorer countries where gender inequality is marked. WHO and the United Nations Joint Programme on HIV/AIDS (UNAIDS) have strongly supported its use.[40] Launched in Britain as early as 1992, the female condom had been supplied by mid-1998 to public sector organisations in 23 countries in Africa, Asia and the Pacific, the Caribbean and Latin America, as well as Europe.[41] More importantly, perhaps, it is being seen as useful in the struggle to contain HIV/AIDS in Africa. In April 1998, UNAIDS convened a meeting of 15 countries intended to accelerate introduction of the female condom in Southern and Eastern Africa: marketing programmes exist (or are planned) in Zimbabwe, Zambia, South Africa, Uganda, Tanzania, and Côte d'Ivoire. Peter Piot, Executive Director of UNAIDS, noted: "UNAIDS undertook to support the female condom sales program because it felt there was a need for a practical means of protecting women from STIs and HIV/AIDS, especially in the developing world. The success of the program and the general growth in use of the female condom is gratifying".[42]

Conclusion

A number of factors have promoted use of the modern condom: a rising living standard from the nineteenth century in Europe and Europe overseas began to create mass markets as well as the desire to limit family size; technological innovation enabled production of the rubber, the latex, and, more recently, the polyurethane condom; mass education created a growing audience for the information offered by the modern birth control movement; the wish of governments in two world wars to protect the health of troops led to further popularisation of the condom as a disease preventive, and as a contraceptive; the new behaviours carried over into civilian life; from the early twentieth century, (non-commercial) nonmarital sex became more widespread as women's sexual behaviour became more like that of men; finally, the advent of HIV/AIDS raised the status of the simple condom to that of a life-saving device, and governments around the globe (some more quickly than others) encouraged the use of condoms as a matter of national policy.

Working against the trend toward greater use have been the continuing association of the device with illicit sex and the unacceptability of contraception to pronatalists. Another retarding force has been individual rejection of the condom as unaesthetic or unreliable. It remains to be seen how far the new female condom, which offers women the personal control over both fertility and disease threats that men through the male condom have enjoyed for some time, will significantly extend the empire of the condom.

References

1 Himes NE. Medical history of contraception. Baltimore: Williams and Wilkins, 1936.
2 Youssef H. The history of the condom. *J Roy Soc Med* 1993 April; **86**: 226–8.
3 McLaren A. *A history of contraception: from antiquity to the present day.* Oxford: Blackwell, 1992.
4 Van Gulik RH. *Sexual life in ancient China.* Leiden: EJ Brill, 1961.
5 Langley LL, ed. *Contraception.* Stroudsburg: Dowden, Hutchinson and Ross, 1973.
6 Fryer P. *The birth controllers.* London: Secker and Warburg, 1965.
7 Dingwall EJ. Early contraceptive sheaths. *BMJ* 1953 Jan; **1**: 40–1.
8 Bernstein EL. Who was Condom? *Hum Fertil* 1940 Dec; **5**(6): 172–86.
9 Pottle FA, ed. *Boswell's London Journal* 1762–1763. London: William Heinemann, 1950.
10 Huxley J. Material of early contraceptive sheaths. *BMJ* 1957 March; **1**: 581–2.
11 Riddle JM. *Eve's herbs. A history of contraception and abortion in the West.* Cambridge: Harvard University Press, 1997.
12 Quiggan P. *No rising generation. Women and fertility in late nineteenth century Australia.* Canberra: Department of Demography, Research School of Social Sciences, Australian National University, 1988.
13 Ball J. Birth control. Practice and attitudes in New South Wales at the turn of the century. BA Hons. thesis, Australian National University, 1975.
14 Caldwell JC and Ware H. The evolution of family planning in Australia. *Popul Stud* 1973 March; **27**(1): 7–32.
15 Report of Royal Commission on the decline of the birth-rate and on the mortality of infants in New South Wales, Vol 2. Sydney: Government Printer, 1904.
16 Davenport-Hines R. Sex, death and punishment. Attitudes to sex and sexuality in Britain since the Renaissance. London: Collins, 1990.
17 Murphy JS. *The condom industry in the United States.* Jefferson: McFarland and Company, 1990.
18 Johnston M. *Ansell. Portrait of an international company.* Melbourne: Campbell Public Relations, 1990.
19 Gordon L. *Woman's body, woman's right. A social history of birth control in America.* New York: Grossman Publishers, 1976.
20 Lewis M. *Thorns on the rose. The history of sexually transmitted diseases in Australia in international perspective.* Canberra: Australian Government Publishing Service, 1998.

21 Brandt AM. *No magic bullet. A social history of venereal disease in the United States since 1880.* New York: Oxford University Press, 1985.
22 Oriel JD. *The scars of Venus. A history of venereology.* London: Springer-Verlag, 1994.
23 Royal Commission on venereal diseases. Final report of the Commissioners. London: HMSO, 1916.
24 Santow G. Trends in contraception and sterilization in Australia. *Austral New Zeal J Obstet Gynaecol* 1991 Aug; **31**(3): 201–8.
25 Gerofi J. A report in the public interest for the SUPRA sex education committee. Sydney: Sydney University Postgraduate Representative Association, 1973.
26 Donovan B, Richters J, Gerofi J. A pharmacopoeia of Australian condoms. *Venereology* 1991 Aug; 4(3): 88–95.
27 Orme A. *Therapeutic goods and HIV/AIDS: quality and availability of condoms, HIV test kits, needles and syringes.* Canberra: Department of Health, Housing and Community Services, 1992.
28 Valderserri RO. Cum hastis sic clypeatis: the turbulent history of the condom. *Bull New York Acad Med* 1988 April; **64**(3): 237–45.
29 Economist Intelligence Unit Retail Business 1995 Feb; **444**: 106–31.
30 Machan D. Condom king. *Forbes* 1995 July; **156**(2): 47.
31 Johnson AM, Wodsworth J, Wellings K, Field J, Bradshaw S. *Sexual attitudes and lifestyles.* Oxford: Blackwell Scientific, 1994.
32 Greer G. *Sex and destiny. The politics of human fertility.* New York: Harper and Row, 1984.
33 Report on interregional workshop on condom services and promotion. Manila: Regional Office for Western Pacific of WHO, 1990.
34 Jones GW, Sulistyaningsih E, Hull TH. Prostitution in Indonesia. Canberra: Research School of Social Sciences, Australian National University, 1995.
35 Mann J, Tarantola DJM, Netter TW. AIDS in the world. *The global AIDS policy coalition.* Cambridge Mass: Harvard University Press, 1992.
36 Chapman S and Hodgson J. Showers in raincoats: attitudinal barriers to condom use in high-risk heterosexuals. *Commun Health Stud* 1988; **12**(1): 97–105.
37 Rosenthal D. *Taking a chance on love: sexual health in the 1990s.* Melbourne: La Trobe University, 1993.
38 Harcourt C and Philpot R. Female prostitutes, AIDS, drugs, and alcohol in New South Wales. In: Plant M, ed. *AIDS, drugs and prostitution.* London: Routledge, 1990.
39 Harcourt C. Prostitution and public health in the era of AIDS. In: Perkins R, Prestage G, Sharp R, Lovejoy F, eds. *Sex work sex workers in Australia.* Sydney: UNSW Press, 1994.
40 www.femalehealth.com/international_publicsector_z.htm (accessed 12 Jun 1998).
41 www.femalehealth.com/intldistr.htm (accessed 12 Jun 1998).
42 www.femalehealth.com/update.html (accessed 12 Jun 1998).

2 Latex condom manufacture

JOHN GEROFI

This chapter deals only with the manufacture of male condoms made from natural rubber. Other types of condom include: male condoms made from plastic materials; female condoms; "natural" condoms made from animal intestines.

These others make up a very small proportion of total condom sales (less than 1 per cent). Plastic male and female condoms may be made of a number of compounds, of which polyurethane is the most common. Styrene ethylene butylene styrene is another material used. Most are dipped on moulds. "Natural" condoms are actually made from the caeca of New Zealand lambs.

Location of factories

Condom manufacture is a very specialised activity, carried out in about 60 factories around the world. Countries in which there are factories known to the author include: Spain, Germany, Poland, Czech Republic, Russia, China, Taiwan, Japan, South Korea, Vietnam, Thailand, India, Malaysia, Indonesia, USA, Mexico, Brazil, and South Africa. Some other factories, which test and pack condoms bought in bulk, are not included in this list.

In general, there has been a considerable shift in manufacture from the developed countries to Asia and Central America, where labour is cheaper. Factories in the UK, Italy and Australia have closed, and many new ones have opened in Asia. Within the European Union, condom production has ceased in the UK and

Italy, and is now concentrated in Spain and Germany, despite the latter's high wages. Even Korea has felt the pressure of rising wages, and two factories have effectively moved to other countries. The quality of condom products in developing countries varies, but a number of the new factories are able to manufacture very high quality products consistently. Although two factories in the USA have closed in recent years, additional capacity has been provided at one other site, so that significant manufacturing capacity remains in that country.

World production

Total world production of condoms is estimated at between 8 and 10 billion per annum, but there are no formal surveys of capacity or production available.

Varieties

The "basic" model of condom is a cylindrical tube terminating in a thickened bead at the open end. At the closed end the condom is basically hemisperhical, usually with a protruding reservoir, intended to catch the semen.

Variants on the basic design may include:

- Changes to the length and circumference of the condom
- Varying the circumference along the length of the condom (shaped condoms)
- Changing the colour by adding pigments
- Modifying the surface of the condom, by having a patterned mould. This can result in ribbed, dotted or similar textures, or in emblems
- Varying the thickness of the condom
- Varying the nature and quantity of the lubricant on the condom
- Removing the reservoir

Other designs include condoms with applicator devices and condoms with glue inside them, to prevent slippage during use.

The most common condom design is approximately 180 mm long (measured on the parallel part), with a (laid flat) width (semi-circumference) of 52 mm. For some Asian markets, it has been found that a smaller width, normally 49 mm, is more appropriate. There are some 45 mm condoms available, but these are very uncommon. Recently, larger condoms have also become available, with width around 56 to 60 mm. Generally, wider condoms are also longer (over 200 mm), while the narrower ones may be shorter.

The different sizes appear to be necessary so that most of the population can find one size that does not slip and yet is not too tight. However, the different condom sizes tend to be geographically distributed, and there are many countries where effectively only one size is available.

The two principal types of shaped condom are generally called contoured and flared. The contoured condom has a constriction intended to correspond wth the area behind the glans, while the flared variety has a larger width near the closed end, giving room for the glans to move. Other complex variations in circumference may be used in more unusual condoms. The contoured design probably has little practical benefit in use.

Recently, one company started marketing the "Pleasure Plus" condom, which was well accepted in certain small groups of users in the USA, and its breakage and slippage rates appear similar to those of traditional condoms.[1] Fundamentally, this product does not have circular symmetry. It has a bulge on one side near the closed end. The mechanical function of the bulge has not been fully explained, but it has been said that the rubber acts like an artificial foreskin. The design ensures that there must be loose rubber near one side of the glans even if the other side is stretched tight. The loose part is supposed to be on the side near the frenulum. Another such product is the "inSpiral". These products are very difficult to remove from the moulds during manufacture and testing. It is likely that a flared condom would have largely the same effect. On the other hand, the psychological aspects of condom acceptability cannot be ignored, and any innovation that makes condoms more appealing is useful.

Pigments may be added to one or both of the latex dips during production. Well chosen pigments will not harm the physical properties of the condom, and may make it more attractive to the user.

So-called "textured" condoms are produced by using appropriately textured moulds. The effect may vary from the finest lines (or even a floral design) to significantly raised lumps on the surface. The more pronounced the texture, the more likely that it will be the site of some form of weakness. Generally, the most skilled manufacturers can make relatively pronounced textures successfully, but most others cannot. Thus use of textured condoms should involve more careful selection of manufacturers and more vigilant testing of the product.

The thickness of condoms can be varied by altering the water content and viscosity of the compounded latex, and the way in which the formers are dipped in latex. Thin condoms are promoted as being extra-sensitive in use, and therefore desirable. Most manufacturers are now producing "regular" condoms with average thickness of approximately 0.07 mm. If the thickness drops below about 0.06 mm, there may be difficulties in meeting the requirements of standards on a consistent basis. A few manufacturers, notably those in Japan, produce a lot of thin condoms, and can do so relatively successfully. Generally, the thinnest condoms currently made are around 0.04 mm thick. Thinner products were previously available, but appear to have been discontinued because of the requirements of international standards and the use of condoms to prevent HIV transmission.

Thicker condoms can be produced more easily than thin ones. They have become popular in a small segment of the market, as being suitable for HIV prevention in anal use. In Europe, these products may legally be labelled "extra-strength" if they meet certain breaking force requirements. Whether the additional thickness really reduces the breakage rate has yet to be determined, and the clinical evidence currently available does not support the requirement. Newer proposals, being incorporated in the 1999 draft joint ISO/EN standard have a burst pressure requirement for extra-strength, but even this has scant clinical support.

A wide range of substances have been applied to condoms as they are being packed. Most still have a powder and a lubricant applied. Currently, three powders are still acceptable: cornstarch, silica, and magnesium carbonate. Talc and lycopodium powder have been shown to be harmful, and most manufacturers have stopped using them.

Silicone fluids are the most commonly used lubricants. Commonly, the viscosity will be between 100 and 350 centistokes, and manufacturers generally apply between 100 and 500 mg to each condom. (The viscosity can be regarded as a measure of the ease with which a fluid flows.) As a result of recent litigation regarding silicone fluids in breast implants, there may be some concerns about further use of the compounds on condoms. Unfortunately, there are no readily apparent substitutes that do not harm rubber.

There are also some other lubricants used, such as the propylene and ethylene glycols, and until recently, an aqueous lubricant. These are much less popular than silicone fluids, except perhaps in the USA.

Spermicidal lubricants are popular in some markets. The most common spermicide used is nonoxynol-9, a surfactant. Other spermicides include nonoxynol-11 and benzalkonium chloride. These spermicides do not mix readily with silicone fluids, and most manufacturers find it easier to mix them with the glycols. Spermicidal lubricants may interfere with the integrity of the package. Frequent, prolonged, contact with the skin, vagina or penis may cause irritation. Higher concentrations are more likely to cause problems than lower ones. The additional protection provided by the spermicide has not been quantified in clinical trials, and sex-workers using condoms on a daily or more frequent basis may find the problems exceed the potential benefits.[2] In any case, there are now reports that spermicide use is associated with urinary tract infections.[3]

The reservoir on the end of a condom is an innovation some decades old. It was promoted as being there to catch the semen after ejaculation. Reservoir-ended condoms may also be a little easier to produce. Plain ended condoms simply require a hemispherical end on the mould. Plain-ended condoms are believed by some to be more suitable for use in anal sex, although the clinical evidence for that is not adequate.

Main raw material

Natural rubber comes from the sap of a tree - *Hevea Brasiliensis*. As the name implies, the species is native to Brazil, but ironically today even the Brazilian condom factories import their latex from Asia. Other varieties, notably *H. Benthamiana*, can also produce rubber, but not in the same quantity and purity as *H. Brasiliensis*.

In Brazil, the trees grow in jungle conditions, and are tapped by local residents. In 1873, to overcome supply shortages, seeds were sent to England, and eventually to Sri Lanka, where the first successful plantations were established. Since then, plantations have spread to Malaysia, Thailand, Indonesia, India, Vietnam and West Africa. They tend to grow best in slightly elevated tropical conditions. Plantation rubber was first marketed in quantity around 1910.

The tree is tapped by cutting a groove like a coarse screw-thread around the bark and placing a cup at the bottom of the groove (see Figure 2.1). Latex is collected daily from the trees, and taken to a central processing area. Some chemicals, such as

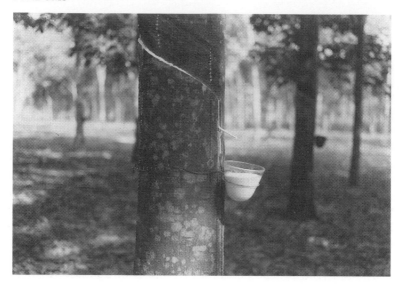

Figure 2.1   Collecting sap from the *Hevea Brasiliensis* tree.
Source: Rubber Institute of Malaysia, Kuala Lumpur.

antifungals and zinc oxide are added after tapping, if the highest quality of latex is required.

At the plantation's central processing area, most of the latex is coagulated and dried for use in rubber tyres and similar articles. A small percentage ends up as liquid latex, which is used for condoms, medical and household gloves, balloons, and similar products that are dipped from the latex. Latex is prepared by adding ammonia (an anticoagulant), a mechanical stabiliser, and antibacterial and antifungal agents. The latex is centrifuged to attain the right solids content (about 60 per cent) and then sent to the condom factories. For condoms, only the highest quality latex, prepared with the maximum care, can be used.

Compounding and vulcanisation

The latex that arrives at the condom factory is essentially a colloidal suspension of the principal constituent – poly-isoprene – in water, with potassium laurate and ammonia. There are also other residual products from the tree, notably proteins.

This latex, basically concentrated from the tree, if solidified, produces an interesting substance, which bounces, and which was originally sought-after in Europe as a pencil eraser. It is, however, neither very strong, nor stable with temperature.

In 1839, Charles Goodyear began experimenting with ways of cooking rubber that led to the discovery of vulcanisation in the 1840s. Vulcanisation is further polymerisation of the isoprene molecules, principally through links with sulphur atoms. The process cross-links the poly-isoprene chains to one another, which gives rubber strength and relative thermal stability.

Rubber condoms became available around the 1870s, and were apparently cast to size for the customer. The process became automated, based on dissolving solid rubber in a solvent (e.g. naphtha) and dipping formers in it. These condoms were thicker than the condoms we know today, and were generally advertised as re-usable. In the 1930s, the present method of dipping directly in an aqueous suspension concentrated from the natural product began to be used.

In modern condom manufacture, a blend of chemicals is made and added to the rubber. It includes:

• Sulphur – the vulcanising agent
• Zinc oxide – which helps initiate the reaction
• One or more accelerators
• A stabiliser – such as potassium laurate
• Possibly an antioxidant
• A pigment – if the condoms are to be coloured.

Other ingredients proprietary to each manufacturer may be added. After mixing the compounded latex must be matured for some time under controlled conditions, during which it is vulcanised to varying degrees, depending on the process.

Dipping

The most significant part of condom manufacture is the dipping operation. Condoms are made by dipping moulds (often called formers) into the compounded latex. The formers are mounted on an endless chain loop, and circulate through the plant. They are usually made of glass, but may also be ceramic. At the start (or end) of the process, the formers are cleaned, using detergent/water sprays and mechanical action. Some plants also have acid/base washes.

After washing, the formers are dried, then dipped into the first vat of latex, which is kept at about 20–25°C. The formers move

25

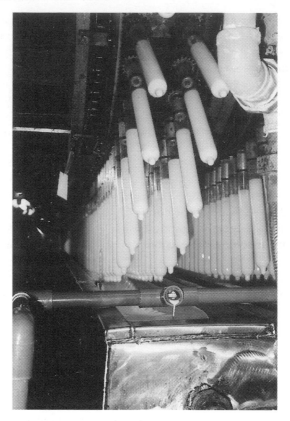

Figure 2.2   Latex condoms emerging from a dripping tank in the factory.
Source: Seohung Industrial Company.

through the dip tank, rise and then go into a heated drying chamber. After drying, they go into the second dip, and after that, are again dried. (A few machines use a third dip.) The bead is formed on the open end by rollers that run on an angle beside the formers.

Depending on the design of the plant, varying degrees of vulcanisation may be carried out in a tunnel oven on the production line. The condoms are removed from the production line by water jets or by rollers. Those needing further vulcanisation or drying are tumbled in large industrial drying machines like clothes dryers.

At some point after bead rolling and drying, either on the production line or off it, the condoms will be washed (leached). This may be done either in a step intended solely for that purpose, or as part of the removal from the dipping line, transport from the dipping line, or wet electronic testing. The degree of washing affects the smell of the product and the level of residual proteins, which can cause allergies.

Testing, quality control, and quality assurance

Quality control tests are conducted on the product during the manufacturing process. Every condom made is tested for leaks before packing. There are two tests, known in the industry as "wet" or "dry".

The wet test measures electrical conductivity between the inside and the outside of the condom. Condoms are put on metal moulds, like the formers, mounted on a chain rather like that on the dipping machine. The condoms are then dipped in a conductive solution, and the resistance between the solution and the mould is measured. Those with low resistance are rejected. The accepted condoms are then dried and rolled off the tester by brushes. The test is usually conducted at less than 100 volts.

The dry test relies on dielectric breakdown. The condoms are mounted on rotating metal moulds, and a conductive rubber flap or metal mesh passes over them. If there is a hole, or a very thin spot, the gap breaks down, and a hole is burned in the condom. These machines operate at between 1200 and 1700 volts.

Condoms with holes are automatically segregated from the other condoms in both designs. The most appropriate choice of testing machine depends on many factors.

Most companies have some level of in-process quality control. This may involve selecting samples at various stages in the process, and subjecting them to various tests, mainly the freedom from holes and inflation tests to the appropriate standards. Some chemical tests may also be done on the dipped product, and some checks may be done on the latex. Poor results or significant trends in sentinel values signal the need for immediate remedial action.

Also, quality assurance testing should be carried out on the packed, finished product, to ensure that the product conforms to the purchaser's (and/or regulatory) requirements. Such testing should also discover serious damage to the product due to malfunction of the packing machines. One of the tests is a sample test for holes, in addition to the screening on the production line. Acceptance testing should be conducted on key raw materials, but many manufacturers rely on the suppliers' specifications.

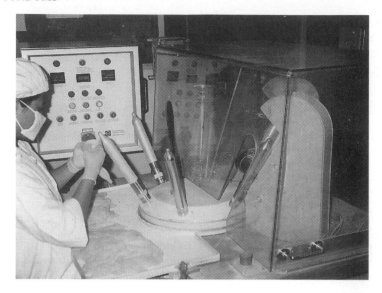

Figure 2.3   Dry high voltage testing machines for latex condoms.
Source: Seohung Industrial Company.

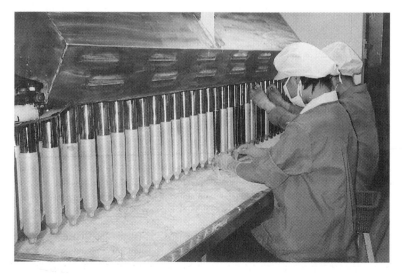

Figure 2.4   Condoms being loaded on metal mandrels for wet electrical testing.
Source: Seohung Industrial Company.

Lubrication and packing

Although packing machines for condoms are generally purpose built, either by specialised manufacturers or by the condom manufacturers themselves, there is nothing unique about them. Generally, they use a laminated foil material, with an inner layer of polyethylene. (Some resin coatings may also provide a heat seal as an alternative to the inner plastic film.) Two rolls of the material are usually used, and they are brought above and below the condom.

Most condoms are now sold with a lubricant on them. The lubricant is most commonly added on the packing machine, just before the pack is heat-sealed. Another method of lubrication is to tumble the condoms in a cylinder of lubricant before they are put on the packing machine.

Different laminated foils may be used for packing. The most effective protection to the condom is afforded by a layer of aluminium foil, at least 8 microns thick. Usually, there is a layer of cellophane or plastic material bonded to the outside of the aluminium, to carry the artwork and statutory information, but also to enhance the strength.

Laminates which do not have an oxygen-impervious layer will give inferior protection against oxidation. Nonetheless, such laminates may be adequate in temperate climates. Some manufacturers use transparent packs, to show off the colours of the condoms. Such transparent materials need to be chosen carefully, to ensure that they block UV radiation and, in hotter climates, are oxygen-impermeable.

The rectangular packs use considerably less packing material than the square ones, and are thus much cheaper. However, it appears that the complex distortions introduced by the rectangular packs may compromise the shelf-life of the product.

Some innovative suppliers have attempted to facilitate the donning of the condom by packing it with an unrolling device. The Topaz is one example. This has a ring packed on the rolled condom. The user pushes down on the ring, which is supposed to unroll the condom as it moves down the penis. The ring has a weak point which can snap during the unrolling, to ensure that it will go over a wide range of penile circumferences and tapers. None of these devices has achieved widespread popularity in the market.

The testing and packing of condoms is the most labour-intensive part of the production process. Many of the surviving factories in the developed world have reduced their labour costs in this part of the production by automation. Some factories have completely automated the operations of foiling, lubrication, packing in consumer packs, and wrapping in shipping cartons. There are also devices available that automatically load the testing machines, although these are not common.

The foiled product may be packed in a "consumer pack" for retail sale, and/or in packs of 100 or one gross.

Regulation

There are two elements to regulation of quality of condoms: (1) requiring the product itself to comply with appropriate product standards; (2) requiring the circumstances under which the product is manufactured to comply with appropriate standards or practices.

The first country to regulate condom quality was Sweden, starting in 1950.[4] The Swedes introduced import controls, requiring each lot of condoms imported into the country to be tested for holes and air inflation; other Scandinavian countries followed. In the USA, the FDA published test requirements for holes in the 1950s, but a national standard only appeared in the 1970s.

Elsewhere, condoms were still taboo in many respects, and were made in factories that were never built or run with the same attention to quality as one expected in the pharmaceutical industry. Throughout the 1970s and 1980s, there was a steady increase in awareness of condom quality issues, culminating in the issue of the ISO standard for condoms in 1990.[5] Many countries began to require that the condoms conform to standards.

Apart from Sweden, a number of other countries successfully controlled the quality of condoms by requiring independent tests on each lot produced (or imported into the country). Other countries had regulations requiring conformance with standards, but enforced them less rigorously, by random market uplifts, or not at all.

The stringency of standards varies. Some countries have resisted the inclusion of the inflation test, and some, e.g. South Africa, still did not require it in 1997. Some countries simply have laxer requirements. For example, in 1997, Hungary still allowed ten times as many holes as the current ISO standard, and had no inflation requirements.[6] Some countries have no standards or regulations at all.

30

Generally, however, increasingly stringent standards have been set, based on laboratory tests, and many manufacturers have been able to meet them. It is not clear, however, what proportion of the world's manufacturers are able to meet consistently the latest (1996) ISO and EN requirements. Additional requirements are likely to be imposed in the future joint ISO/EN standard.

Some countries required compliance with Good Manufacturing Practices (GMP), which are a general code of practice for manufacturers of medical devices. These were virtually subsumed by the more general ISO 9000 series of standards,[7] which describe a model for quality management, intended to be applicable to all industry and commerce. More recently, additional standards have been published on the application of the ISO 9000 series to quality of medical devices. In the European Union, the way in which factories must demonstrate compliance with GMP and product standards is dictated by the Medical Device Directive.[8]

The two principal elements of a regulatory system are enforcement of the product standard and enforcement of GMP. The latter involves the checking of record keeping, factory organisation and consistency of practices. Both arms can be enforced with varying rigour. Sweden regulated condom quality successfully simply by an initial type test, plus testing every lot against a product standard. Other countries concentrate on GMP and do only rare product tests. GMP is intended to ensure that good quality is built into the product, rather than weeding out bad lots. While the lot-by-lot testing of delivered condoms does fulfil the latter function, it also makes the manufacturer aware that poor quality product will most likely be rejected.

There has been growing emphasis in recent years on GMP, mostly using the ISO 9000 series of standards, and variants of them, specifically designed for medical devices. Manufacturers can have voluntary certification that they meet these requirements, or in some jurisdictions, certification may be mandatory. It involves independent audits.

Tests have shown that factories with GMP certification do not necessarily produce good condoms. Also a factory may have intrinsic GMP without being certified. Thus, GMP is only one component in ensuring good quality product is delivered, and alone, should not be taken as evidence that the product is acceptable. Unfortunately, many regulatory authorities place excessive faith in auditing and GMP documentation as a means of ensuring condom quality.

Acknowledgements

Valuable comments on the text were provided by Gavin Shaw.

References

1 Trussell J, Warner D L, Hatcher RA. Condom slippage and breakage rates. *Fam Plann Perspect* 1992; **24**: 20.
2 American Health Consultants. No added STD protection from spermicidal condoms. *Contracept Technol Update*, 8 Aug 1998; **19**: 105–6.
3 Fihn S D, Boyko E J, Normand E H, Yarbro P, Scholes D. Use of spermicide-coated condoms and other risk factors for urinary tract infection caused by *Staphylococcus saprophyticus. Arch Int Med* 9 Feb 1998; **158**(3): 281–7.
4 Linde S. Inspection and control of contraceptives at apotekens celtrallaboratorium. *Sartyck ur Svensk Farmaceutisk Tidschrift*, 1973; 77: 588–594.
5 ISO 4074 – 1990 (several parts). Rubber condoms. Geneva: International Organisation for Standardisation, 1990 (later revised in 1996).
6 (Hungarian condom standard) Gumi Óvszer, Egészségüyi Ágazati Szabvány, MSZ-03, Magyar Szabványügyi Hivatal, 1979.
7 ISO 9001. Quality systems – model for quality assurance in design, production, installation and servicing. Geneva: International Organisation for Standardisation, 1994.
8 Official Journal of the European Communities, L169, Volume 36, 12 July, 1993.

3 International quality standards: unfinished evolution

PHILIP KESTELMAN

Used properly, good quality rubber condoms are 99 per cent effective against conception and sexually transmitted infections (STIs), with a first year method pregnancy rate of 2 per cent. Combining a condom with a separate, vaginal spermicide is as effective as the Combined Pill, with a pregnancy rate of 0.1 per cent.[1] The combination of Condom-cum-Spermicide is arguably 99.9 per cent effective for STI prophylaxis.

In typical use, condoms (like oral contraceptives) prove less effective and the main source of condom "failure" is simply non-use by nominal users. Hence the paramount importance of easing personal motivation to use condoms properly: sound information (including simple instructions); and a range of choice among brands.

In descending order of gravity, the principal causes of condom failure in practice are: breakage; slippage; and leakage. Nonetheless, slippage occurs mainly through neglecting the single most important instruction: **during withdrawal after ejaculation, hold the rim of the condom to the base of the penis**.

Both objectively and subjectively, condom *breakage* during coition is by far the worst eventuality, afflicting under 1 per cent of good quality condoms, used carefully. Thus condom *strength* is essential; and in particular, freedom from local *weakness* (notably at the closed end).

Prescribing condom integrity is the primary justification for a *standard*, whose implementation should minimise condom failure. According to the last British Standard[2], "the only feasible way of establishing compliance of condoms with the requirements of this standard is by inference from determinations of the properties of a sample of condoms taken from a large population". Hence the need for sample-testing every batch of condoms, packaged as supplied to consumers (inside individual containers, e.g. foils).

Differences between national standards imply the desirability of a common, International Standard, under the auspices of the International Organization for Standardization (ISO). Following a proposal by the Swedish ISO member-body, an ISO Technical Committee on Mechanical Contraceptives (ISO/TC 157) met six times between 1975 and 1989.

Stimulated by the rise of HIV/AIDS, the world's first International Condom Standard (ISO 4074) was completed in 1990.[3] The first European Standard (EN 600: 1996)[4] was based on ISO 4074, which was revised[5] in 1996. (ISO 4074–1: 1996 is summarily compared with EN 600: 1996 in Appendix A).

Also based on ISO 4074, the World Health Organization (WHO) condom *Specification* includes contractual elements.[6] ISO/TC 157 is now drafting a harmonised, global condom standard (EN ISO 4074).

This chapter focuses on ISO 4074, mentioning other relevant standards and the prospective EN ISO 4074. The relationship between condom standards and reliability (safety) is discussed critically.

At the outset, it is important to distinguish between 100 per cent electrical *screening* (so-called "electronic testing") of condoms, and batch *sample-testing*. Before packaging, condoms are screened for holes and thin spots: in the *dry* state, at high voltage; and/or in the *wet* state, at low voltage: eliminating conductive speciments (see Chapter 2).

From each batch of packaged condoms (typically 1000 gross, or 144 000), under 1 per cent are sampled randomly for testing against a standard. Sample-testing thus checks both electrical screening and any subsequent damage from the packaging process – which involves the proximity of heat, pressure, sharp edges and machine oil.

Currently in separate parts, ISO 4074 prescribes condom sampling requirements, test methods and physical properties: dimensions (length and width); leakage (water-tested); strength (air-tested); packaging and labelling. Tolerances for batch defectiveness are also prescribed: Acceptable Quality Levels (AQLs) of about 1 per cent (see Appendix B).

34

Dimensions

Like other bodily dimensions, penile length and girth vary widely. It is important that the condom fits comfortably and that the rim can be held to the base of the penis during withdrawal after ejaculation.

Length

Excluding any teat (reservoir), ISO 4074–1: 1996 prescribes a condom minimum length of 160 mm; while EN 600: 1996 requires a minimum length of 170 mm. ISO 4074 constrains minimum *individual* length (160 mm), permitting 1 out of 13 shorter specimens (AQL = 4.0 per cent),[5] necessitating an average length of at least 170 mm.

On the other hand, EN 600 only prescribes minimum *average* length (for 10 condoms per batch).[4] EN ISO 4074 may permit none out of 13 specimens under 160 mm long (AQL = 1.0 per cent: see Appendix B).

Width

Condom size refers primarily to perimeter (twice flat width). For cylindrical (parallel-sided) condoms, width can be measured anywhere. However, shaped condom perimeter varies along the length (for example, narrowing and/or widening near the closed end). Where then should width be measured for sizing purposes?

The condom must grip the penile base, near the rim. Accordingly, ISO 4074 prescribes width measured 25–35 mm from the rim, permitting 1 out of 13 specimens over 2 mm outside nominal width (AQL = 4.0 per cent).[5]

Less rationally, EN 600 prescribes midbody width (55–85 mm from the rim), only requiring an average (for 10 condoms per batch) within 2 mm of nominal width (44–56 mm), marked on the packet.[4] EN ISO 4074 may permit none out of 13 specimens, measured at the narrowest section within 35 mm of the rim, over 2 mm outside nominal width.

WHO specifies parallel-sided, teat-ended, smooth, colourless, odourless, and tasteless condoms.[6] However, there is no evidence that plain-ended (teatless) condoms are more vulnerable to breakage in use.

Thickness

Rubber thickness varies along the condom length, usually increasing from the rim towards the closed end, and average thickness ranges narrowly (about 0.06–0.07 mm) between most brands. The USA Condom Standard prescribes a minimum average thickness of 0.03 mm, permitting 1 out of 13 thinner specimens (AQL = 4.0 per cent).[7]

On grounds of comfort and strength, WHO also prescribes a mean condom thickness (measured near the closed end, near the rim and midbody), permitting none of 13 specimens outside the range 0.05–0.08 mm.[6] However, neither ISO 4074 nor EN 600 prescribes thickness.

EN 600 prescribes a minimum tensile (midbody) breaking force for "extra-strong" brands much higher than for ordinary condoms, necessitating rubber over 0.09 mm thick. Ultra-thin condoms (under about 0.04 mm thick) are constrained by air-bursting requirements (see below).

Difficult to measure directly, condom thickness at different sections may be calculated simply by weighing cylinders (20 mm long) of measured width. Then, assuming a rubber density of 0.933 g/cm^3,

$$\text{mean thickness (mm)} = 0.0268 \times \frac{\text{Mass (mg)}}{\text{Width (mm)}}$$

EN ISO 7074 may describe this gravimetric method of determining condom thickness.

Aqueous leakage

Applied to every batch imported since 1959, the pioneering, Swedish Condom Standard prescribed sample-testing for holes by filling each specimen with 300 ml (0.3 litre) of water; suspension for three minutes; inspection for visible leakage; and rolling on absorbent paper, darkened by leakage through invisible holes (See Figure 3.1). Out of 300 specimens tested, four were allowed to leak: a requirement failed by every single condom brand sample-tested in 1963 by the British consumer-body.[8]

The first British Standard (BS 3704: 1964) prescribed testing condoms for holes by filling with 300 ml (half a pint) of water; suspending freely (without supporting the closed end) for three

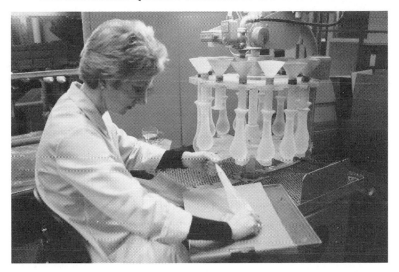

Figure 3.1   Low volume (300 ml) water testing for condom leakage.
Source: *Which? Way to Health*, August 1993, reproduced with permission
of the Consumers' Association, London.

minutes; and inspection for visible leakage.[9] BS 3704 prescribed a
1.0 per cent cumulative tolerance for condoms leaking water;
reduced to 0.5 per cent in 1972, when holes were detected
more sensitively (with rolling, as in Sweden).

ISO 4074–5: 1980 (Testing for holes) originally prescribed
suspending each 300 ml water-filled specimen for one minute;
rolling on absorbent paper; and inspection for leakage over
25 mm from the rim. The sensitivity of this method varied widely
between testing laboratories. Accordingly, the Second Edition
(ISO 4074–5: 1984) prescribed only suspending water-filled
specimens; and inspection for leakage within 125 mm of the
closed end.[10]

ISO 4074–1: 1990 prescribed an AQL of 0.4 per cent[3] for
condoms with holes, visibly leaking water during suspension,
within 125 mm of the closed end. Referring to the same method,
while evaluating holes over 25 mm from the rim, the 1995 WHO
Specification prescribed an AQL of 0.25 per cent.[6]

The USA Condom Standard also manages without absorbent
paper, ignoring holes within 25 mm of the rim, with an AQL of 0.4
per cent.[7] More rationally, the US Food and Drug Administration
prescribes: suspending each water-filled condom freely; rolling on

absorbent paper, standing the condom on its closed end; and evaluating leakage within 140 mm of the closed end.[11] (Compare air-testing within 150 mm of the closed end: see below.)

ISO 4074–1: 1996 (with ISO 4074–5: 1996)[5,12] now prescribes an AQL of 0.25 per cent for condoms with visible holes, or leaking water (during suspension or rolling, over 25 mm from the rim). Prescribing the same AQL for condoms with holes, EN 600: 1996 describes alternative test-methods: either 300 ml water-testing (as ISO 4074–5: 1996)[12]; or electrical testing (similar to wet "electronic testing", i.e. 100 per cent screening).[4]

EN 600 electrical testing involves filling each specimen with about 200 ml aqueous saline (1.0 per cent NaCl); immersion in saline (25 mm below the rim) for 10 seconds; measuring condom resistance; and checking any low resistance (below 2 megohm) by water-testing. EN ISO 4074 may permit either water-testing or electrical/water-testing for condom leakage.

Carey et al.[13] reported leakage of HIV-sized microspheres (0.1 micron in diameter) through a substantial minority of condoms satisfying water-testing, but estimated that the efficacy of such condoms exceeded 99.99 per cent. Herman et al.[14] reckoned that condom water-testing detected holes of diameter exceeding 7–140 micron, depending on rubber wettability.

Freely suspending a condom, filled with 300 ml of water, exerts a maximum axial force – or *thrust* – of only 3 newton: less than ordinarily strenuous coition. Holes at the closed end are detected relatively insensitively during both suspension and horizontal rolling. Considering the methodological ebb and flow since 1980, and the lack of clinical validation, the salience of most holes, only detectable on absorbent paper, may well be doubted.

Apart from condoms with visible holes, EN ISO 4074 may introduce an AQL of 1.0 per cent for condoms with serious *visible defects*: broken, missing or severely distorted rims; or permanent adhesions. In 1975–96, BS 3704 prescribed an AQL of 0.4 per cent for specimens with *any* visible defect, including embedded foreign matter, oily dirt, surplus rubber, bubbles, and abrasions.[2]

For condoms with serious visible defects, an AQL of 1.0 per cent now appears oddly lax. An AQL of 0.4 per cent would be more satisfactory for condoms with holes or serious visible defects.

Strength

In practice, the ultimate catastrophe is condom breakage, especially during coition. Good quality rubber is a necessary but insufficient condition of strong condoms, which may incorporate local weaknesses.

Tensile properties

Minimum tensile properties characterise good quality rubber. Condom tensile testing involves: cutting a midbody collar, a cylindrical test-piece 20 mm long; measuring its thickness and flat width; looping it over parallel rollers 15 mm in diameter; separating the rollers, thereby stretching the test-piece radially; and measuring its breaking extension and force (see Figure 3.2).

ISO 4074–1: 1990 originally permitted 1 defective out of 20 test-pieces (an AQL of 2.5 per cent): under a breaking elongation of 650 per cent (stretching the test-piece to 7.5 times its initial girth). The same AQL was prescribed for test-piece breakage under a force of 30 newton, implying a midbody thrust of about 75 newton: (like a 7.5 kg weight); and for tensile strength under 17 MPa (about 170 kg/cm^2 unstretched cross-section).[3]

EN 600: 1996 prescribes a *median* breaking elongation exceeding 700 per cent for 13 midbody test-pieces per batch. It also requires a test-piece median breaking force exceeding 39 newton for ordinary condoms; or 100 newton for nominally "extra-strong" brands.[4] (The same tensile requirements are prescribed after condom oven-treatment at 70°C for two days).

Such minimum tensile properties may appear formidable. However, tensile testing addresses only a few *midbody* sections which, protected inside the rolled condom, may not typify the more vulnerable closed end. Moreover, only typical (average or median) tensile properties are evaluated.

Gerofi et al.[15] concluded that tensile properties were unrelated to condom breakage in use; and ISO 4074 and WHO no longer prescribe tensile requirements.[5,6] Nonetheless, EN ISO 4074 may prescribe a minimum average tensile breaking force (100 newton) for nominally "extra strong" condoms.

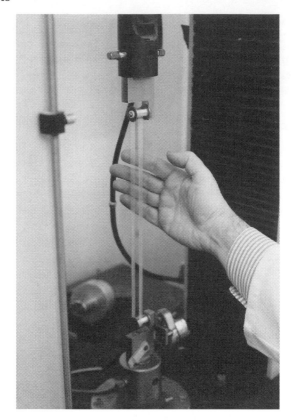

Figure 3.2 Tensile testing for midbody mean strength.
Source: *Which? Way to Health*, August 1993, reproduced with permission of the Consumers' Association, London.

Air inflation

Compared to tensile testing, air testing (as shown in Figure 3.3) challenges the strength of a much larger proportion of the whole condom; and with a far larger sample size. The Swedish Condom Standard (1959) prescribed a minimum average bursting volume of 25 litres (for 100 condoms per batch), with a maximum Relative Standard Deviation (Coefficient of Variation) of 25 per cent, permitting about 1 per cent of condoms below 10 litres.

ISO 4074–1: 1990 originally prescribed an AQL of 1.5 per cent for condoms bursting under an excess pressure of 0.9 kPa, (under 1 per cent of atmospheric pressure); and the same AQL

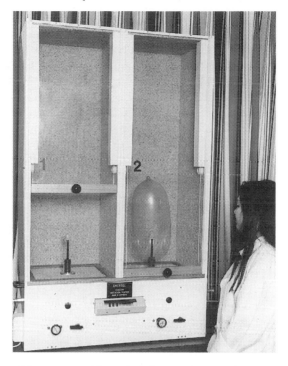

Figure 3.3   Air testing for condom weakness.

for condoms below a volume of 15 litres (for condoms of typical, nominal width 52 mm).[3] Air-testing involves fixing each specimen 150 mm from the closed end before inflation (as described in ISO 4074–6: 1996).[16]

ISO 4074–1: 1996 now prescribes an air-tested AQL of 1.0 per cent, allowing five defectives out of 200 specimens (see Appendix B): condoms visibly leaking air, or bursting under minimum pressure (1.0 kPa); with the same AQL for condoms leaking visibly, or bursting under minimum volume (16 litre for condoms of average, midbody width 52 mm: proportional to width squared).[5]

ISO 4074 prescribes the same minimum bursting properties and AQL after condom oven-treatment at 70°C for seven days.[5,19] Requiring air-testing before *and* after oven-treatment makes ISO 4074 the highest condom standard in the world.

EN 600: 1996 prescribes an AQL of 1.5 per cent for condoms visibly leaking air, or bursting under 1.0 kPa and/or 18 litre.[4] EN

41

ISO 4074 may prescribe a minimum pressure of 1.0 kPa for ordinary condoms; and a higher minimum pressure of 1.5 kPa for "extra-strong" brands, exerting midbody thrusts of around 30 and 45 newton, respectively. (Minimum volumes of 16–18 litre may depend on width.)

Considering that condom breakage in use is far worse than most leakage, it may be wondered why air-tested condom weakness enjoys such a high tolerance (an AQL of 1.5 per cent being six times the AQL of 0.25 per cent for water-tested leakage). Moreover, there is no clinical basis for a fixed minimum bursting volume as high as 18 litres. So why not fix a lower tolerance for condoms visibly leaking air, or bursting under lower minimum pressure or volume (say, AQL = 0.4 per cent for specimens below 0.9 kPa and/or 12 litres, exerting a minimum thrust of 20 newtons more than ordinary coition)?

Free et al.[17] air-tested a field-aged batch of exceptionally weak condoms, of which nearly half (49 per cent) broke in use; and 37 per cent air-burst under 5 litres. However, only 7 per cent of used, unbroken condoms burst under 5 litres, implying that weaker specimens rarely survive coition intact.

Most condoms thicken towards the closed end, which therefore inflates last, like toy balloons; and minimum bursting volume leaves that critical area under-stressed. Even at a volume of 18 litre, condom strain (stretch) remains below 100 per cent at the closed end, but over 500 per cent near the fixture.[18] Thus air-tested defectiveness proves a surrogate for closed end weakness.

Opinion remains divided on whether to evaluate condoms visibly leaking air as defective (as in ISO 4074–1: 1996 and EN 600: 1996).[4,5] The current USA Standard ignores and replaces specimens leaking air, arguing that leakage is already detected aqueously (see above).[7]

Condom air-testing probably detects midbody holes of initial diameter over 20 micron. However, at the under-strained closed end, air inflation may only find holes of uninflated diameter over 100 microns (0.1 mm), again inverting clinical priorities.

In view of the closed end problem, an ISO/TC 157 Working Group on Condom Bursting Properties is considering air-testing a shorter condom length (even 50 mm: one-third of the current 150 mm), or constraining inflation to proceed from the closed end.

Water inflation

Water-testing for leakage involves low volume (0.3 litre) water inflation; and a typical condom supports at leat 20 times that volume (over 6 litre). Indeed, it may be wondered why condoms are not tested for leakage with at least 500 ml of water, merely doubling any hole diameter.

The British Standard originally prescribed a *bursting strength* test: filling a hole-free, 300 ml water-tested specimen with 3 litres of water.[9] However, this condom was not suspended freely, its closed end resting on a platform, 400 mm below the rim.

A potential solution to the closed end problem therefore lies in freely suspending condoms, filled with some minimum volume of water (around 2 litre, depending on condom inflatable mass, for an AQL of 1.0 per cent). Exploratory research during the 1980s, under the auspices of ISO/TC 157, appeared promising; and condom water inflation effectively overstresses the closed end bi-axially, much like coition.

Packaging and labelling

ISO 4074 and EN 600 require each rolled condom to be packaged inside an individual container (hermetically sealed foil). In addition, EN 600 prescribes an outer packet (consumer package).[4] Neither ISO 4074 nor WHO insists upon a consumer package.

WHO prescribes individual container shape (square), material (metal/plastic) and impermeability; and dressing material quantity.[6] EN ISO 4074 may prescribe test methods – without requirements – for individual container integrity, and for measuring total dressing material (not only the lubricant on the condom, of primary interest to consumers).

ISO 4074 prescribes individual container expiry-dating[7]; required by EN 600 within five years of manufacture (and on the consumer package)[4]. However, predicting condom shelf-life remains highly controversial.

Both ISO 4074 and EN 600 imply that condom oven-treatment (so-called "artificially accelerated ageing") simulates normal storage conditions. However, EN ISO 4074 may caution that, while disclosing major formulation or vulcanisation errors, batch-sampled condom oven-treatment provides no information on shelf-life.

Among other details on the consumer package, both ISO 4074 and EN 600 prescribe instructions for condom storage, use and disposal. Not conspicuously user-friendly, EN ISO 4074 may prescribe similar instructions. (See also Chapter 14).

Neither ISO 4074 nor EN 600, apart from nominally "extra-strong" brands, challenges any labelling claim or implication of exceptional safety. EN ISO 4074 may prescribe consumer package labelling of width, but not of thickness or strength.

The US Food and Drug Administration recently prohibited labelling rubber devices as "hypo-allergenic", a claim misleadingly based upon testing for sensitivity to residual process chemicals, not to rubber proteins.[20] Rubber condoms must now be labelled prominently: "**Caution: This Product Contains Natural Rubber Latex Which May Cause Allergic Reactions.**"

Conclusions

An ideal condom is an *acceptable* condom; users have diverse preferences; and standards should not compromise brand choice unreasonably, e.g. by discouraging thinner brands. Well informed about condom brands, consumers need protecting against relatively weak specimens. They need to know: how to use the condom; its width (size) and thickness (or weight); and its strength – whether "ultra-thin", ordinary or "extra-strong". An ideal standard both protects and informs consumers.

Between 1964 and 1989, British Standards Institution certification (Kitemarking) involved batchwise cumulative sample-testing requirements. Obligatory in Europe on packets of condoms manufactured since mid-1998, CE-marking guarantees neither quality nor reliability. For sustained consumer protection, the forthcoming EN ISO 4074 will need rigorous implementation by sample-testing every batch of packaged condoms.

The current ISO 4074 is the world's highest condom standard. Whether EN ISO 4074 will raise or lower that standard remains to be seen.

Clinical validation of ISO 4074 is not in prospect; and without challenging condom integrity where it matters most – at the closed end – EN ISO 4074 will remain a surrogate for good quality. Nonetheless, condom quality has improved over the past 30 years, and modern condoms are safer than ever before.

References

1 Kestelman P, Trussell J. Efficacy of the simultaneous use of condoms and spermicides. *Fam Plann Perspect* 1991; **23**: 226–7.

2 British Standards Institution. *British Standard Specification for Natural rubber latex condoms.* BS 3704: 1989. London: BSI, 1989.

3 International Organization for Standardization. International Standard ISO 4074–1: 1990 *Rubber condoms – Part 1: Requirements – Condoms in consumer packages.* Geneva: ISO, 1990.

4 Comité Européen de Normalisation. European Standard EN 600: 1996 *Natural rubber latex male condoms.* Brussels: CEN, 1996.

5 International Organization for Standardization. International Standard ISO 4074–1: 1996 *Rubber condoms – Part 1: Requirements.* Geneva: ISO, 1996.

6 World Health Organization/Joint United Nations Programme on HIV/AIDS. *The Male Latex Condom: Specification and Guidelines for Condom Procurement.* Geneva: WHO/UNAIDS, 1998.

7 American Society for Testing and Materials. *Standard Specification for Rubber Contraceptives (Male Condoms)* D 3492–96. Philadelphia: ASTM, 1996.

8 Consumers' Association. *Contraceptives. Which?* Supplement. London: CA, 1963.

9 British Standards Institution. *British Standard Specification for Rubber Condoms.* BS 3704: 1964. London: BSI, 1964.

10 International Organization for Standardization. International Standard ISO 4074–5: 1984 *Rubber condoms – Part 1: Testing for holes.* Geneva: ISO, 1984.

11 Pierdominici VJB Jr. *et al.* Water leak testing of male latex condoms. *Lab Inform Bull 3970.* Winchester: US Food and Drug Administration, 1995.

12 International Organization for Standardization. International Standard ISO 4074–5: 1996 *Rubber condoms – Part 5: Testing for holes – Water leak test.* Geneva: ISO, 1996.

13 Carey RF *et al.* Effectiveness of latex condoms as a barrier to human immunodeficiency virus-sized particles under conditions of simulated use. *Sex Trans Dis* 1992; **19**: 230–4.

14 Herman BA *et al.* Sensitivity of water leak tests for latex condoms. *J Test Eval* 1993; **21**: 124–8.

15 Gerofi J *et al.* A study of the relationship between tensile testing of condoms and breakage in use. *Contraception* 1991; **43**: 177–85.

16 International Organization for Standardization. International Standard ISO 4074–6: 1996 *Rubber condoms – Part 6: Determination of bursting volume and pressure.* Geneva: ISO, 1996.

17 Free MJ *et al.* An assessment of burst strength distribution data for monitoring quality of condom stocks in developing countries. *Contraception* 1986; **33**: 285–99.

18 Gerofi JP and Shelley GA. Condom inflation testing: strain distribution during test. *J Test Eval* 1991; **19**: 244–9.

19 International Organization for Standardization. International Standard ISO 4074–7: 1996 *Rubber condoms – Part 7: Oven conditioning.* Geneva: ISO, 1996.

20 US Food and Drug Administration. Natural rubber-containing medical devices: user labelling. *Federal Register* 1997; **62**: 51021–30.

4 Contraceptive efficacy of the male condom

JAMES TRUSSELL

Four pieces of information about contraceptive efficacy would help couples to make an informed decision when choosing a contraceptive method.

- *Pregnancy rates during typical use* show how effective the different methods are during actual use (including inconsistent *or* incorrect use).
- *Pregnancy rates during perfect use* show how effective methods can be, where perfect use is defined as following the directions for use; for barrier methods, perfect use means correctly *using* the method at every act of intercourse.
- *Pregnancy rates during imperfect use* show how ineffective methods will be if they are used incorrectly or inconsistently.
- *The percentage of perfect users* or percentage of cycles during which a method is used perfectly reveals how hard it is to use a method correctly and consistently.

The difference between pregnancy rates during imperfect use and pregnancy rates during perfect use reveals how forgiving of imperfect use a method is. The difference between pregnancy rates during typical use and pregnancy rates during perfect use reveals the consequences of imperfect use. This difference depends both on how unforgiving of imperfect use a method is and on how hard it is to use that method perfectly.

In this chapter, we review methods for measuring contraceptive efficacy during typical and perfect use and review studies published in English of contraceptive efficacy of the male condom in developed countries. All studies were conducted in the United States unless otherwise noted in the text and tables.

Survey data limitations

Information on efficacy during typical use of the male condom is available from survey data (particularly the National Surveys of Family Growth (NSFG) in the United States). Data from nationally representative surveys have the advantage of pertaining (in theory) to the actual population of users of each method, but they suffer from the disadvantage of reporting errors, especially since efficacy information is obtained from retrospective reports of contraceptive use and contraceptive failures. The most serious defect is under-reporting of abortion. Estimates of the extent of under-reporting can be obtained by comparing the number of abortions derived from surveys of abortion providers conducted by The Alan Guttmacher Institute with the number reported in the NSFG. The overall level of abortion under-reporting in the 1995 NSFG for the four-year period 1991–4 is estimated to be 55 per cent in the main interview, 48 per cent in the computer-assisted self-interview for sensitive topics, and 41 per cent where the main interview is combined with the self-report.[1] It is likely that some induced abortions are misreported as spontaneous abortions,[2] but the sum of reported-induced and spontaneous abortions is without doubt too low. The consequence, *ceteris paribus*, is an under-reporting of contraceptive failure. It is likely that what appears in some instances to be continuous use of a contraceptive method in fact contains a contraceptive failure, or that what appears to be a simple switch of methods in fact resulted from contraceptive failure. Although attempts have been made to correct for such under-reporting in prior NSFGs by using surveys of abortion patients to ascertain contraceptive use prior to the abortion,[3] the correction for under-reporting of abortion produces estimates of contraceptive failure that are probably too high because women in abortion clinics over-report use of a contraceptive method at the time they became pregnant.[4] Moreover, it seems likely that women in personal interviews for the NSFG also would tend to over-report use of a contraceptive method at the time of a reported conception. Evidence for this suspicion is provided by a first-year probability of pregnancy of 6 per cent for the IUD (a method with little scope for user error) among married women in the 1976 and 1982 NSFGs. This probability is much higher than rates observed in clinical trials of IUDs.[5] We would naturally expect over-reporting of contraceptive method use in both the NSFG and in surveys conducted in abortion clinics: responsibility for the pregnancy is shifted from the woman (or couple) to the method.[4]

Information from well-supervised clinical trials is also subject to potential bias because it is plausible that subjects may alter their behaviour while they know that they are being observed, so that efficacy results during typical use may not be generalisable beyond the trial conditions. Specifically, subjects may be more likely to use a contraceptive method perfectly either to please the investigator or to avoid embarrassment or even possible censure when the investigator discovers imperfect use. However, given the high levels of imperfect use reported in well-supervised trials,[6–10] it is not at all evident that the Hawthorne effect is important.[a,11] Nevertheless, subjects in a clinical trial are certainly not a random sample of all actual or potential users of the method(s) being studied; they themselves choose to be in a clinical study and they must meet the selection criteria established by the investigators (e.g. have a history of normal menstrual cycles, have frequent coitus, have no known impairment to fecundity).

Measuring contraceptive efficacy

Two methods are used in the literature to measure contraceptive efficacy. The oldest is the Pearl index,[12] which is computed as 100 times the ratio of pregnancies to exposure measured in woman-years: $PI = 100(P/E)$, where P and E are the number of pregnancies and number of woman-years of exposure, respectively. If exposure is originally tallied in cycles instead of calendar months, then woman-years is computed as the number of cycles divided by 13 (not 12). It is a common mistake to assume that the Pearl index falls between 0 (if nobody became pregnant) and 100 (if everybody became pregnant). Instead, the maximum value is not 100 but 1200 (or 1300 if exposure is tallied in cycles), which would occur if each woman became pregnant in her first month

---

[a] The Hawthorne effect refers to the impact on research outcomes caused by subjects' reactions to being observed. The name derives from a series of experiments conducted between 1924 and 1932 at the Hawthorne Works of the General Electric Company. A surprising outcome from several of these experiments was that even adverse changes in work conditions (such as dramatically reducing workspace illumination) resulted in increased work productivity.[11]

(cycle) in the study; the value for chance or no method would be typically about 250 among young married women. Data on the Hutterites, an Anabaptist sect that does not practise birth control, yield a 12-month Pearl index of 254.[13] Despite the fact that the index is easy to misinterpret, it is attractive because it is easy to compute. However, it is seriously flawed as a summary measure of contraceptive failure because pregnancy rates typically decline with duration of use.

A decline could arise for two reasons. First, the risk of contraceptive failure could be identical across women but decline with use as couples learn how to achieve correct technique every time. Learning-by-doing may occur, but it would seem more likely for methods like the condom, diaphragm, cervical cap, or periodic abstinence than for methods like the pill or IUD. Second, the risk of contraceptive failure could be constant over time for each woman but vary across women. The most likely circumstance is that, while both factors operate, learning-by-doing is relatively unimportant and the decline is caused mainly because those most prone to become pregnant do so early, leaving a pool increasingly dominated by the most conscientious or least fecund users. As a consequence, the longer one runs a study, the lower will be the overall pregnancy rate if each woman is allowed to contribute her total exposure to the analysis.[14]

For example, the Pearl pregnancy rate for couples using the condom to prevent any further pregnancies based on the 1973 National Survey of Family Growth (NSFG) would be 7.5 if each woman were allowed to contribute a maximum of 12 months of exposure and 2.8 if women could contribute a maximum of 60 months.[15] Which rate is correct? Of course, both are correct, but they clearly measure different things. Comparing results from different studies with different maximum durations of exposure is virtually meaningless, because failure is measured with a rubber yardstick. This problem is so serious that Sheps[16] has concluded that the index "cannot be said to estimate any quantity of interest or to be a meaningful approach to the comparison of several groups".

This problem is eliminated by the use of life table procedures, in which a separate pregnancy rate for each month is calculated; the complements of these rates are then chained together to yield the cumulative proportion conceiving within x months.[17] Investigators commonly report 12-month probabilities of contraceptive failure, and they also occasionally report 6-, 18-, or 24-month probabilities. Such probabilities are certainly easy to interpret. For example, the 1995 NSFG revealed that of 100 women who started to use the male condom and who continued to use it unless they failed, 9 became accidentally pregnant within one year.[2]

Measuring contraceptive efficacy during perfect use

Many investigators have recognized the importance of distinguishing between contraceptive failure associated with user error and failure attributable to the inherent inadequacy of the method itself. By convention, all pregnancies that occur in a menstrual cycle in which a method is used imperfectly are labelled user pregnancies. Only those pregnancies that occur during a cycle during which a method is used perfectly are classified as method pregnancies; *perfect use* does not imply that the method does not fail, only that the method is used consistently and correctly according to a well-specified set of rules. There is no problem with this convention, although not all pregnancies classified as user failures will in fact be user failures. In a cycle in which a method is not used or is used incorrectly during some acts of intercourse but used correctly during other acts, then a resulting pregnancy could be due to method failure rather than user error.

Until recently, when computing separate *method* and *user* pregnancy rates (pregnancies divided by exposure), investigators included all cycles of exposure in the denominator of *both* method *and* user failure rates. Under this convention, the sum of method and user failure rates is the overall or total pregnancy rate. The common misinterpretation was that the resulting method pregnancy rate yields information about the inherent efficacy of the method. That this interpretation is incorrect is obvious when one realizes that inherent method efficacy can be measured only when the numerator (method failures) is assessed in relation to the proper risk set (exposure only when the method is used perfectly). Method failure rates computed by this incorrect procedure confound inherent method efficacy with the proportion of exposure that is characterised by perfect use. This error was quite widespread; method (or theoretical) failure rates have almost always been calculated incorrectly, because investigators remove only the pregnancies attributable to improper use from the analysis, although they retain all exposure. For example, among the twelve clinical trials of periodic abstinence reviewed by Trussell and

Kost,[5] "method only" calculations (all incorrect) were found in nine.[8]

The following simple example illustrates the logical error in the old procedure for computing method and user failure rates. Suppose that there are two method pregnancies (that occurred during perfect use) and eight user pregnancies (that occurred during imperfect use) during 100 women-years of exposure to the risk of pregnancy. Then the traditional calculation is that the user pregnancy rate is 8 per cent and the method of pregnancy rate is 2 per cent; the sum of the two is the overall failure rate of 10 per cent. By convention, however, method pregnancies can occur only during perfect use, and by definition user pregnancies cannot occur during perfect use. If there are 50 years of perfect and 50 years of imperfect use in the total of 100 years of exposure, then the method pregnancy rate would be 4 per cent and the user pregnancy rate would be 16 per cent.

Correctly computed estimates of the risk of pregnancy during correct and consistent use of the cervical cap,[9,18] sponge,[9,18] diaphragm[9,10] female condom,[18,19] male condom,[10] and ovulation method of periodic abstinence[8,20] are now available from clinical trials, and the US Food and Drug Administration requires that a table providing estimates of the risk of pregnancy during both perfect and typical use be included in the package labelling of all contraceptives marketed in the United States. The current version of that table is reproduced here as Table 4.1; a detailed explanation for the derivation of these estimates is provided elsewhere.[4]

Studies of contraceptive efficacy of the male condom

We identified 15 published studies of the contraceptive efficacy of the male condom, results from these studies are summarised in Table 4.2.[2,3,10,21–32] Nine of these studies are based on retrospective reports of women in sample surveys.[2,3,22,27–32] Results from these population-based surveys are simply not comparable with results from a carefully designed and executed prospective clinical trial because the research designs are so different. The estimate of the probability of pregnancy during the first year of typical use of the male condom shown in Table 4.1 is the average of results for married women in the 1976 and 1982 National Surveys of Family Growth (NSFG) uncorrected for under-reporting of abortion[5] and for all women in the 1988 NSFG corrected for

Table 4.1 Percentage of women experiencing an unintended pregnancy during the first year of typical use and the first year of perfect use of contraception and the percentage continuing use at the end of the first year: United States*

Method	% of women experiencing an unintended pregnancy within the first year of use		% of women continuing use at 1 year[c]
	Typical use[a]	Perfect use[b]	
Chance[d]	85	85	–
Spermicides[e]	26	6	40
Periodic abstinence	25		63
Calendar	–	9	–
Ovulation method	–	3	–
Sympto-thermal[f]	–	2	–
Post-ovulation	–	1	–
Cap[g]			
Parous women	40	26	42
Nulliparous women	20	9	56
Sponge			
Parous women	40	20	42
Nulliparous women	20	9	56
Diaphragm[g]	20	6	56
Withdrawal	19	4	–
Condom[h]			
Female (Reality)	21	5	56
Male	14	3	61
Pill	5		71
Progestin only	–	0.5	–
Combined	–	0.1	–
IUD			
Progesterone T	2.0	1.5	81
Copper T 380A	0.8	0.6	78
LNg 20	0.1	0.1	81
Depo-Provera	0.3	0.3	70
Norplant and Norplant-2	0.05	0.05	88
Female sterilisation	0.5	0.5	100
Male sterilization	0.15	0.10	100

Emergency Contraceptive Pills: Treatment initiated within 72 hours after unprotected intercourse reduces the risk of pregnancy by at least 75%.[i]
Lactational Amenorrhea Method: LAM is a highly effective, *temporary* method of contraception.[j]
* Source: Trussell, Table 31-1.[4]

[a] Among *typical* couples who initiate use of a method (not necessarily for the first time), the percentage who experience an accidental pregnancy during the first year if they do not stop use for any other reason.
[b] Among couples who initiate use of a method (not necessarily for the first time) and who use it *perfectly* (both consistently and correctly), the percentage who experience an accidental pregnancy during the first year if they do not stop use for any other reason.

[c] Among couples attempting to avoid pregnancy, the percentage who continue to use a method for one year.

[d] The percentages becoming pregnant in columns 2 and 3 are based on data from populations where contraception is not used and from women who cease using contraception in order to become pregnant. Among such populations, about 89% become pregnant within one year. This estimate was lowered slightly (to 85%) to represent the per cent who would become pregnant within one year among women now relying on reversible methods of contraception if they abandoned contraception altogether.

[e] Foams, creams, gels, vaginal suppositories, and vaginal film.

[f] Cervical mucus (ovulation) method supplemented by calendar in the pre-ovulatory and basal body temperature in the post-ovulatory phases.

[g] With spermicidal cream or jelly.

[h] Without spermicides.

[i] The treatment schedule is one dose within 72 hours after unprotected intercourse, and a second dose 12 hours after the first dose. The Food and Drug Administration has declared the following brands of oral contraceptives to be safe and effective for emergency contraception: Ovral (1 dose is 2 white pills), Alesse (1 dose is 5 pink pills), Nordette or Levlen (1 dose is 4 light-orange pills), Lo/Ovral (1 dose is 4 white pills), Triphasil or Tri-Levlen (1 dose is 4 yellow pills).

[j] However, to maintain effective protection against pregnancy, another method of contraception must be used as soon as menstruation resumes, the frequency or duration of breast-feeding is reduced, bottle feeding is introduced, or the baby reaches six months of age.

under-reporting of abortion.[3] As stated above, we suspect that contraceptive failure rates based on the NSFG alone would tend to be too low because induced abortions (and contraceptive failures leading to induced abortions) are under-reported but would tend to be too high because contraceptive failures leading to live births are over-reported. These two sources of bias would tend to cancel, whereas adjustment for under-reporting of induced abortion would make the pregnancy rates too high. However, we would expect estimates based only on married women from the 1976 and 1982 NSFGs to be underestimates of the risk of pregnancy for all women, since unmarried women regularly having intercourse experience higher pregnancy rates during typical use of contraceptives than do married women.[3] We conclude that the estimates based on the experience of married women in the 1976 and 1982 NSGFs uncorrected for under-reporting of abortion are likely to be too low and that those based on the experience of all women in the 1988 NSFG corrected for under-reporting of abortion are likely to be too high; our final estimate is the average of these two.

Two of the six remaining studies are not based on clinical trials. John[25] interviewed three groups in Shepshead, England – (1) a random sample of married women in the town's only clinical practice, (2) all women who attended the family planning clinic

Table 4.2 Summary of studies of contraceptive failure of the male condom[a]

Reference	N for Analysis	Risk of Pregnancy					Characteristics of the sample[w]	LFU (%)[g]	Comments
		Life-table 12-month percentage pregnant	Pearl Index Pregancy Rate						
			Index	Total exposure	Maximum exposure				
Potts and McDevitt, 1975[20]	397	2.1[b]					77% males age 40; all married	4.8[c]	Britain; postal trial of spermicidal lubricated condom
Peel, 1972[21]	96		3.9	3689 mo	60 mo		All married	2.9[t]	Britain; Hull Family Survey
Glass et al., 1974[22]	2057	4.2					All white; at recruitment aged 25–39 and married; at enrollment, all women had been using the diaphragm, IUD, or pill successfully for at least 5 months	<1.0[v]	Britain; Oxford/FPA study
Vessey et al., 1988[23]	?		4.4	10 000[c] yr	24 mo		All white; at recruitment aged 25–39 and married; at enrollment, all women had been using the diaphragm, IUD, or pill successfully for at least 5 months	?	Britain; Oxford/FPA study

Table 4.2 (continued)

Reference	N for Analysis	Risk of Pregnancy				Characteristics of the sample[w]	LFU (%)[g]	Comments
		Life-table 12-month percentage pregnant	Pearl Index Pregancy Rate					
			Index	Total exposure	Maximum exposure			
Nelson et al., 1997[10]	383	5.0[d]				14% aged < 21, 77% aged 21–34, 8% aged 35–; 69% living with partner; 44% nulligravid[t]	4.6[c,d,g]	Avanti plastic condom; random assignment to Avanti plastic or Ramses latex condom
John, 1973[24]	85		5.7[c]	261 yr	>7 yr	?	?	Britain; retrospective study
Vessey et al., 1982[25]	?		6.0	4317 yr	24 mo	All white and aged 25–34; all married at recruitment; at enrollment all women had been using the diaphragm, IUD, or pill successfully for at least 5 months	0.3[t,v]	Britain; Oxford/FPA study
Nelson et al. 1997[10]	384	6.4[d]				14% aged <21, 77% aged 21–34, 8% aged 35+; 69% living with partner; 44% nulligravid[t]	4.7[c,d,g]	Ramses latex condom; random assignment to Ramses latex or Avanti plastic condom
Jones and Forrest, 1992[3]	1728	7.2				Aged 15–44[t]	21[r]	NSFG 1988; probability when standardised and corrected for estimated under-reporting of abortion = 15.8[s]

Bracher and Santow, 1992[26]	262	8.1	16% aged <20; 65% aged 20–29; 19% aged 30+; 48% parity 0; 83% married or cohabiting	25[r]	Australian Family Survey; first use of method
Trussell and Vaughan, 1998[2]	2925	8.7	Aged 15–44[t]	21.4[r]	NSFG 1995
Schirm et al., 1982[27]	1223	9.6[s]	Aged 15–44; all married[t]	18.2[r]	NSFG 1973 and 1976
Grady et al., 1983[28]	1223	9.7[s,c]	Aged 15–44; all married[t]	18.2[r]	NSFG 1973 and 1976
Vaughan et al., 1977[29]	696	10.1[s]	Aged 15–44; all married[t]	19.0[r]	NSFG 1973
Grady et al., 1986[30]	526	13.8[s]	Aged 15–44; all married[t]	20.6[r]	NSFG 1982
Westoff et al., 1961[31]	~212	13.8c 10 062 mo ?	All married	5.7[r]	FGMA study

Source: Trussell,[4] Table 31-9.

a Updated from Trussell and Kost,[5] Table 6.

b 24-month probability; 12-month probability not published.

c Calculated by James Trussell from data in the article.

d 6-month probability; 12-month probability not available.

g Most of these studies incorrectly report the loss to follow-up probability (LFU) as the number of women lost at any time during the study divided by the total number of women entering the study. Thus, these are the probabilities presented in the table. However, the correct measure of LFU would be a gross life-table probability. When available, gross 12-month probabilities are denoted by the letter "g".

r Nonresponse rate for entire survey.

s Standardised: Vaughan et al.[29] (1973 NSFG) – intention (the average of probabilities for preventers and delayers); Grady et al.[28] (1973, and 1976 NSFG) – intention (our calculation: the average of probabilities for preventers and delayers); Schirm et al.[27] (1973 and 1976 NSFG) – intention, age and income; Grady et al.[30] (1982 NSFG) – intention, age, poverty status, and parity; Jones and Forrest[3] (1988 NSFG) – duration, age, marital status, poverty status.

t Total for all methods in the study.

v The authors report that LFU for "relevant reasons" (withdrawl of cooperation or loss of contact") was 0.3% per year on average; if 0.3% are LFU per year, then 2.8% would be LFU in 9.5 years. In the 1982 study, women had been followed for 9.5 years. LFU including death and emigration is about twice as high as LFU for "relevant reasons".

w Unless otherwise noted, characteristics refer to females.

in the town during a one-year period, and (3) all women in the town whose pregnancy ended in a birth or an induced abortion during that year – to obtain their retrospective reports of contraceptive experience. Potts and McDevitt[21] assessed the efficacy of spermicidally lubricated condoms by recruiting a sample of condom users from the regular mail-order customers at the Marie Stopes Memorial Centre. Prospective male participants were asked to use the new condom exclusively for a period of two years and to complete a questionnaire after two years of use. The results are very difficult to generalise to the larger population of condom users, for several reasons. The sample of males was rather old – 77 per cent were aged 40 or over, 51 per cent were aged 45 or over, and 24 per cent were aged 50 or older – and so might be expected to have low coital frequency, giving the decline in coital frequency with age.[33] Many of their female partners, being about two years younger, would be well past the age of peak fecundity. Finally, only pregnancies leading to a live birth were counted as failures. Note that this is the only study of the contraceptive efficacy of spermicidally lubricated condoms published in the literature.

Three of the remaining four studies are all based on the same prospective clinical trial (the Oxford/FPA study).[33,34,26] At recruitment, all women were required to be married and aged 25–39 and to have been using the diaphragm, pill, or IUD successfully for at least five months. The last criterion ensures that the sample is self-selected for better-than-average contraceptive use or lower-than-average fecundity or coital frequency. Combined with the age criterion, the sample of eventual condom users also would be expected to have lower-than-average coital frequency.

The remaining study is the only clinical trial of the efficacy of the male condom conducted according to modern standards of design, execution, and analysis.[10] Couples were randomly assigned to use either a latex condom or a polyurethane condom for seven months. Adjusted for the use of emergency contraceptive pills, the six-cycle probability of pregnancy during consistent use of the latex condom was 1.2 per cent. Assuming a constant per-cycle probability of pregnancy, the 13-cycle probability of pregnancy during consistent use would be 2.6 per cent, and this is the estimate shown in column 3 of Table 4.1. This estimate is consistent with an estimate based on studies of condom breakage and slippage. Under the assumption that 1.5 per cent of condoms break or slip off the penis and that women have intercourse twice a week, then about 1.5 per cent of women would experience condom breaks during the half-week that they are at risk of pregnancy during each cycle. The per-cycle probability of conception would be reduced by 98.5 per cent, from 0.1358 to only 0.0020, if a condom failure results in no protection whatsoever against pregnancy, so that about 2.6 per cent of women would become pregnant each year.[34] Unfortunately, breakages and slippage rates did not accurately predict pregnancy rates during consistent use in the clinical trial of the latex and polyurethane male condom,[10] and estimates of condom breakage and slippage during intercourse or withdrawal vary substantially across studies in developed countries,[35] from a low of 0.6 per cent among commercial sex workers in Nevada's legal brothels[35] to a high of 7.2 per cent among monogamous couples in North Carolina.[36]

Conclusion

There is only one clinical study of the contraceptive efficacy of the male condom that meets modern standards of design, execution, and analysis. Therefore, the knowledge base for assessing the contraceptive efficacy of the male condom during perfect use is very limited. Unfortunately, it has not yet proved possible to predict contraceptive efficacy during perfect use from far less costly clinical studies of slippage and breakage. There is no randomised clinical trial comparing the efficacy of spermicidally lubricated and non-spermicidally lubricated condoms and therefore no empirical (as opposed to mathematical modelling[34]) basis for claims that spermicidally lubricated condoms provide better protection against pregnancy, or indeed whether they have any effects other than raising the price[37] and raising the risk of urinary tract infection among women.[38,39]

Evidence about the contraceptive efficacy of the male condom during typical use is based on sample surveys, particularly the National Surveys of Family Growth (NSFG). Analyses of these data suffer from one major limitation. They assume that information is accurately reported in the NSFG, but it is likely both that sensitive behaviours and events – such as induced abortion – may not be completely reported and that other information – such as precisely which methods were used in each month over a period of several years – simply cannot be accurately recalled despite a respondent's best intentions. Moreover, the concept of use is an elastic one that depends entirely on whether a woman considers herself to be a user of a particular method at a specific point in time. The degree to which the results based on the NSFG more or less accurately reflect reality is, therefore, unknowable.

The male condom clearly does not provide perfect protection against pregnancy even when used correctly and consistently. It is equally clear that emergency contraceptive pills can reduce the risk of pregnancy by at least 75 per cent in the event of condom slippage and breakage.[40] Increased knowledge about and availability of emergency contraception could make male condoms a more attractive contraceptive option for those concerned about contraceptive efficacy.

References

1 Fu H, Darroch JE, Henshaw SK, Kolb E. Measuring the extent of abortion underreporting in the 1995 National Survey of Family Growth. *Fam Plann Perspect* 1998, **30**: 128–33, 138.

2 Trussell J, Vaughan B. Contraceptive failure, discontinuation, and resumption of method-related use: results from the 1995 NSFG. *Fam Plann Perspect* 1999; **31**: 64–72, 93.

3 Jones EF, Forrest JD. Contraceptive failure rates based on the 1988 NSFG. *Fam Plann Perspect* 1992; **24**: 12–19.

4 Trussell J. Contraceptive efficacy. In: Hatcher RA, Trussell J, Stewart F *et al.* (eds). *Contraceptive technology: seventeenth revised edition*. New York, NY: Ardent Media, 1998.

5 Trussell J, Kost K. Contraceptive failure in the United States: a critical review of the literature. *Stud Fam Plann* 1987; **18**: 237–83.

6 Farr G, Gabelnick H, Sturgen K, Dorflinger L. Contraceptive efficacy and acceptability of the female condom. *Am J Public Health* 1994; **84**: 1960–4.

7 Richwald GA, Greenland S, Gerber MM, Potik R, Kersey L, Comas MA. Effectiveness of the cavity-rim cervical cap: results of a large clinical study. *Obstet Gynecol* 1989; **74**: 143–8.

8 Trussell J, Grummer-Strawn L. Contraceptive failure of the ovulation method of periodic abstinence. *Fam Plann Perspect* 1990; **22**: 65–75.

9 Trussell J, Strickler J, Vaughan B. Contraceptive efficacy of the diaphragm, the sponge and the cervical cap. *Fam Plann Perspect* 1993; **25**: 100–5, 135.

10 Nelson A, Bernstein GS, Frezieres R, Walsh T, Clark V, Coulson A. Study of the efficacy, acceptability and safety of a non-latex (polyurethane) male condom. N01-HD-1-3109. Bethesda MD: National Institutes of Health, 1997.

11 Borgatta EF, Borgatta ML. *Encyclopedia of sociology*. New York NY: MacMillan Publishing, 1992.

12 Pearl R. Factors in human fertility and their statistical evaluation. *Lancet* 1933; **225**: 607–11.

13 Sheps MC. An analysis of reproductive patterns in an American isolate. *Popul Stud* 1965; **19**: 65–80.

14 Potter RG. Length of the observation period as a factor affecting the contraceptive failure rate. *Milbank Mem Fund Q* 1960; **38**: 140–152.

15 Trussell J, Menken J. Life table analysis of contraceptive failure. In: Hermalin AI, Entwisle B (eds). *The role of surveys in the analysis of family planning programs*. Liège, Belgium: Ordina Editions, 1982: 537–71.

16 Sheps MC. Characteristics of a ratio used to estimate failure rates, *Biometrics* 1966; **22**: 310–21.
17 Potter RG. Application of life table techniques to measurement of contraceptive effectiveness. *Demography* 1966; **3**: 297–304.
18 Trussell J, Sturgen K, Strickler J, Dominik R. Comparative contraceptive efficacy of the female condom and other barrier methods. *Fam Plann Perspect* 1994; **26**: 66–72.
19 Farr G, Gabelnick H, Sturgen K, Dorflinger L. Contraceptive efficacy and acceptability of the female condom. *Am J Public Health* 1994; **84**: 1960–4.
20 Trussell J, Grummer-Strawn L. Further analysis of contraceptive failure of the ovulation method of periodic abstinence. *Am J Obstet Gynecol* 1991; **165**: 2054–9.
21 Potts M, McDevitt J. A use-effectiveness trial of spermicidally lubricated condoms. *Contraception* 1975; **11**: 701–10.
22 Peel J. The Hull family survey: II. Family planning in the first five years of marriage. *J Biosoc Sci* 1972; **4**: 333–46.
23 Glass R, Vessey M, Wiggins P. Use-effectiveness of the condom in a selected family planning clinic population in the United Kingdom. *Contraception* 1974; **10**: 591–8.
24 Vessey MP, Villard-Mackintosh L. McPherson K, Yeates D. Factors influencing use-effectiveness of the condom. *Br J Fam Plann* 1988; **14**: 40–3.
25 John APK. Contraception in a practice community. *J R Coll Gen Pract* 1973; **23**: 665–75.
26 Vessey M, Lawless M, Yeates D. Efficacy of different contraceptive methods. *Lancet* 1982; **1**: 841–2.
27 Bracher M, Santow G. Premature discontinuation of contraception in Australia. *Fam Plann Perspect* 1992; **24**: 58–65.
28 Schirm AL, Trussell J, Menken J, Grady WR. Contraceptive failure in the United States: the impact of social, economic, and demographic factors. *Fam Plann Perspect* 1982; **14**: 68–75.
29 Grady WR, Hirsch MB, Keen N, Vaughan B. Contraceptive failure and continuation among married women in the United States, 1970–75. *Stud Fam Plann* 1983; **14**: 9–19.
30 Vaughan B, Trussell J, Menken J, Jones EF. Contraceptive failure among married women in the United States, 1970–73. *Fam Plann Perspect* 1977; **9**: 251–258.
31 Grady WR, Hayward MD, Yagi J. Contraceptive failure in the United States: estimates from the 1982 National Survey of Family Growth. *Fam Plann Perspect* 1986; **18**: 200–9.
32 Westoff CF, Potter RG, Sagi PC, Mishler EG. *Family growth in metropolitan America.* Princeton NJ: Princeton University Press, 1961.
33 Trussell J, Westoff CF. Contraceptive practice and trends in coital frequency. *Fam Plann Perspect* 1980; **12**: 246–9.
34 Kestelman P, Trussell, J. Efficacy of the simultaneous use of condoms and spermicides. *Fam Plann Perspect* 1991; **23**: 226–7, 232.
35 Albert AE, Warner DL, Hatcher RA, Trussell J, Bennett C. Condom use among female commercial sex workers in Nevada's legal brothels. *Am J Public Health* 1995; **85**: 1514–20.
36 Steiner M, Piedrahita C, Glover L, Joanis C. Can condom users likely to experience condom failure be identified? *Fam Plann Perspect* 1993; **25**: 220–3, 226.
37 Roddy RE, Cordero M, Ryan KA, Figueroa J. A randomized controlled trial comparing nonoxynol-9 lubricated condoms with silicone lubricated condoms for prophylaxis. *Sex Trans Inf* 1998; **74**: 116–19.
38 Fihn SD, Boyko EJ, Normand EH *et al.* Association between use of spermicide-coated condoms and *Escherichia coli* urinary tract infection in young women. *Am J Epidemiol* 1996; **144**: 512–20.

39 Fihn SD, Boyko EJ, Chen CL, Normand EH, Yarbro P, Scholes D. Use of spermicide-coated condoms and other risk factors for urinary tract infection caused by *Staphylococcus saprophyticus*. *Arch Intern Med* 1998; **158**: 281–7.
40 Trussell J, Rodríguez G, Ellertson C. Updated estimates of the effectiveness of the Yuzpe regimen of emergency contraception. *Contraception* 1998; **59**: 147–51.

5 Condoms for the prevention of sexually transmitted infections

ADRIAN MINDEL, CLAUDIA ESTCOURT

Condoms offer protection against many sexually transmitted infections (STIs). However, the degree of protection is dependent on reliable and consistent use, on the biological characteristics of the different infections, and on the type of sexual activity. Reliable condom use means using a good quality condom for all genital contact, ensuring the condom remains in place throughout the sexual act and ensuring that the condom does not break or slip off during withdrawal. It is also important to make sure that the outside of the condom is not contaminated with genital secretions.

Condoms offer protection by acting as a barrier to bacteria, viruses and protozoa. There have been several studies that have documented the impervious nature of latex condoms to STIs including HIV, Herpes simplex virus, and chlamydia.[1] Although the integrity of condoms against other microbes has not been tested, it is unlikely that these infective agents would be able to cross the latex barrier.

There are many infections that can be transmitted sexually. However, the exact method of transmission and infectivity of the different STIs determines how effective condoms will be (Table 5.1). For example, those infections transmitted via mainly genital secretions (e.g. gonorrhoea) are likely to be dramatically reduced by the use of condoms. On the other hand, condoms are unlikely to prevent infections transmitted by close bodily contact (e.g. pubic lice) and will only offer limited protection for those infections that involve wide areas of the genitalia and surrounding skin (e.g. genital warts and genital herpes).

Table 5.1   Method of transmission and probability of transmission of various infections

Infection	Method of transmission	Probability of sexual transmission per act of sexual intercourse
Gonorrhoea	Contact with semen or cervical secretions	High
Chlamydia	Contact with semen or cervical secretions	Moderate
Genital mycoplasmas	Contact with semen or cervical secretions	Moderate
Trichomoniasis	Vaginal secretions and possibly semen	Moderate
Non-specific urethritis	Contact with semen or cervical secretions	Moderate
HIV	Contact with semen or cervical secretions or blood	Low
Hepatitis B	Contact with semen or cervical secretions or blood	High
Hepatitis C	Contact with semen or cervical secretions or blood	Very low
CMV	Contact with semen or cervical secretions or urine	High
Genital herpes	Contact with virus from vesicles or blisters or intact skin or mucus membranes	High from lesions; low from intact skin[a]
Human papillomavirus, including genital warts	Contact with genital warts or intact skin or mucus membranes	Moderate[a]
Syphilis	Contact with genital ulcers or lesions of secondary syphilis	High
Chancroid	Contact with genital ulcers	High
Lymphogranuloma venereum	Contact with genital ulcers	High
Donovanosis	Contact with genital ulcers	High
Pubic lice	Close body contact with an infected individual	High[a]
Scabies	Close body contact with an infected individual	High[a]
Molluscum contagiosum	Close body contact with an infected individual	Moderate[a]
Hepatitis A	Faeces	High[b]

[a] These infections can be transmitted by close bodily contact as well as penetrative sexual intercourse. [b] Transmitted via faeco-oral contact not via penetrative sex.

The type of sexual activity will also have an impact on condom efficacy. Condoms are often used for vaginal and anal sex but less often for orogenital sex (fellatio). However, several infections including gonorrhoea, herpes and syphilis can be transmitted by this route.

The efficacy of condoms to prevent STIs has been assessed using a variety of methodologies. These include case control studies, cohort studies and cross-sectional studies. Small sample sizes and different methods for assessing condom use have complicated the interpretation of these studies.

In order to assist with interpretation we have looked at the evidence (where it exists) for each infection. Some studies have pooled data and looked at prevention of STIs in general rather than at specific infections. The HIV pandemic has spawned renewed interest in condoms and a disproportionate amount of recent information relates to this infection.

STIs in general

A large cohort study in Thailand followed 2417 men for an average of 22 months. The relative risk of incident presumptive STIs (i.e. signs and/or symptoms suggestive of STIs without laboratory confirmation) was 6.87 (95 per cent CI 5.07–9.03) in those who never used condoms with female commercial sex workers (CSW), 7.10 (95 per cent CI 5.48–9.20) in those who sometimes used condoms with female CSWs, and 2.28 (95 per cent CI 1.82–2.84) in those who always used condoms with CSWs.[2]

By contrast, a postal survey of 477 female university students in Michigan showed that condom usage was not related to a history of STIs[3] and a cohort study of 598 individuals from two STD clinics in Baltimore suggested that self-reported condom use was not associated with any decreased risk in STIs.[4] However, the methodology of this study may have been flawed and its conclusions biased.[5, 6]

Bacterial infections

Gonorrhoea

Mathematical modelling has suggested that condom use, even by a small proportion of individuals has a dramatic effect on the incidence of gonorrhoea.[7] Barlow published the first evidence that condoms offered protection against gonorrhoea in 1977. He studied male patients who had presented to St Thomas' Hospital London during the first 6 months of 1975. Patients were classified into three groups: "correct" condom users (condoms used throughout each act of sexual intercourse with recent sexual partners), "incorrect" users, and all other attendees. Only 4 per cent of correct users had gonorrhoea compared with 13 per cent of incorrect users and 14 per cent of all other attendees. The difference between correct users the rest of the clinic was significant ($p < 0.001$).[8] A study conducted in males serving in the American Navy in 1977 showed no benefit of condoms,[9] although a subsequent re-analysis suggested a moderate benefit (0/29 condom users vs. 71/499 – 14 per cent non-users developed gonorrhoea, $p < 0.05$).[10] Case control studies have confirmed the protection offered by consistent condom use (OR 0.31 95 per cent CI 0.17 – 0.56),[11] or condom use during the last month (OR 0.68 95 per cent CI 0.44 – 1.06),[12] and a cross-sectional survey from three STD clinics in the USA showed that failure to use condoms was associated with an increased risk of acquiring gonorrhoea (OR 1.38 95 per cent CI 1.03–1.87).[13]

Condoms also offer protection to women. A large study from a public STD clinic in Denver showed that condom users had a 30 per cent reduction in gonorrhoea incidence (adjusted OR 0.61 95 per cent CI 0.05–0.76). However, the authors did not attempt to assess the frequency or adequacy of condom use.[14] A similar result was shown from a study in 435 female commercial sex workers (CSWs) in Peru where consistent condom use was associated with a lower risk for gonorrhoea (OR 0.04 95 per cent CI 0.2–1.00), although this was not statistically significant ($p = 0.07$).[15] Other studies support this effect including those in Australian, Thai, Burmese, Indonesian, Greek, and Dutch female CSWs.[16–19] In the latter study 229 female CSWs were followed from 1986–94. The relative risk (RR) of gonorrhoea in the group that "mainly" used condoms was 3.6 (95 per cent CI 2.4–5.1) compared with 4.8 (95 per cent CI 3.1–7.4) in those that seldom used condoms.[20] Finally a case control study from a STD clinic in Baltimore showed that condom use during the last month reduced the risk of gonorrhoea acquisition (OR 0.4 95 per cent CI 0.19–0.87).[12]

The type of relationship (regular or non-regular) during which condoms are used may have an important bearing on efficacy. This was highlighted in a study of 938 women in London, where consistent condom use with regular partners resulted in a high degree of protection. None of 106 women who always used condoms developed gonorrhoea compared with 1/149 (0.7 per cent) often users, 9/305 (3.0 per cent) occasional users, or 13/376 (3.5 per cent) never users, $p < 0.001$. There was no correlation between condom use with non-regular partners and the proportion with gonorrhoea.[21]

Several studies have assessed the effect of "barrier contraceptives" on gonorrhoea without trying to separate the different techniques. The largest of these studies was conducted in 2247 women attending the Venereal Disease Clinic in Nashville in 1979. The relative risk of acquiring gonorrhoea was 0.11 (CI 0.08–0.17) in those who used barrier contraception (condoms or diaphragms).[22] Similar results were obtained from a study of 2005 women attending a family planning clinic in Louisiana. Gonorrhoea rates in oral contraceptive (o.c.) users was 11.5/100 compared with 9.9/100 in IUD users, and 4.2/100 in women using barrier contraceptives ($p < 0.05$ comparing o.c. users and barrier users, and IUD users and barrier users).[23] Very similar results were obtained from a study in 2 019 women attending a family planning clinic in Louisiana in 1973. The rates of gonorrhoea in oral contraceptive users was 10.6/100 compared with 9.5/100 in IUD users and 1.7/100 in those using barrier contraception (condom–diaphragm–foam) ($p < 0.05$).[24]

Not all studies have confirmed the protective efficacy of condoms. A case control study of women (735 with gonorrhoea and 958 controls) attending the STD clinic in Birmingham, Alabama, suggested that condoms alone did not appear to offer protection for gonorrhoea (adjusted relative risk 0.87 95 per cent CI 0.67–1.1). However, women using condoms as well as spermicides (various types available commercially) had a relative risk of 0.41 95 per cent CI 0.21–0.79).[25]

Chlamydia infection and related conditions

Chlamydiae are obligate intracellular parasites that cause a variety of diseases in humans. *Chlamydia trachomatis* causes genital tract infections. Chlamydial infections are among the commonest STIs worldwide. In men the infection usually presents with urethritis. However, in women the infection is often asymptomatic. Long-term consequences include pelvic inflammatory disease (PID) leading to ectopic pregnancy and infertility and the possibility of spread to the newborn at the time of delivery, resulting in ophthalmia neonatorum and pneumonitis. Chlamydia is transmitted via exchange of body fluids, in particular semen and cervical secretions.

Up until recently, screening for chlamydia has been limited by the need in women for a pelvic examination and in men for a specimen of urethral discharge, and poor sensitivity and specificity of many of the tests. However, the availability of DNA amplification techniques performed on urine specimens has opened the way for large-scale screening and intervention studies.

There are no published prospective cohort or intervention studies to assess the efficacy of condoms for the prevention of chlamydia. However, several cross-sectional and case control studies have been published. The largest of these looked at 13 204 female military recruits in the USA during 1996/7. Nine point two per cent had chlamydia and the adjusted odds ratio for "having had a partner who did not always use a condom" was 1.4 (95 per cent CI 1.1–1.6).[26] A study in Gothenberg using chlamydial culture in 5785 women attending family planning clinics revealed a chlamydial prevalence of 7.3 per cent. The adjusted odds ratio for women using no contraception was 1.9 (95 per cent CI 1.3–3.0) compared with condoms alone.[27]

A study in 229 female CSWs, who were followed from 1986–94, showed that the relative risk of chlamydia in the group that "mainly" used condoms was 2.5 (95 per cent CI 1.6–3.7) compared with 2.1 (95 per cent CI 1.2–3.8) in those who seldom used condoms.[26] In female CSWs in Japan, condom use increased significantly from 6 per cent in 1990–1 to 25 per cent in 1992–3 ($p < 0.002$) and this was mirrored by a reduction in chlamydial detection rates from 16 to 12 per cent ($p < 0.0001$).[28] In Sydney, Australia consistent condom use by local CSWs (i.e. women born in Australia or who spoke English at home) was associated with lower rates of chlamydia than for international CSWs where condom use was low.[16] Mathematical modelling also suggests that condom use even by a minority of individuals will have a dramatic effect on the incidence of chlamydia.[7]

As mentioned above in relation to gonorrhoea, the type of relationship (regular of non-regular) during which condoms are used may have an important bearing on efficacy. Condom use with regular but not with non-regular partners appears to offer some protection against chlamydia.[24]

In males a case control study showed that consistent condom use was negatively associated with chlamydial urethritis (OR 0.67 95 per cent CI 0.44–1.03).[11]

Prior to the availability of sensitive and specific tests for the diagnosis of chlamydia, urethritis was often classified as gonococcal or non-gonococcal urethritis (NGU) with most cases of NGU presumed to be caused by chlamydia. Evidence suggesting that condoms offer protection against NGU is inconclusive.[8] However, condoms appear to offer some protection against non-gonococcal, non-chlamydial urethritis, particularly for consistent users (OR 0.59 95 per cent CI 0.43–0.79).[11]

The role of Mycoplasmas in NGU is still unresolved. None the less, these organisms colonise the genital tract and can be sexually transmitted. Males who consistently use condoms are significantly less likely to be colonised with mycoplasmas than non-users (14 per cent vs. 43 per cent, $p < 0.001$).[29]

Syphilis

Treponema pallidum, the causative organism of syphilis, is an obligate human parasite. The treponemes probably enter the body through micro-abrasions in the epithelium, caused by the trauma of intercourse, and then migrate down into the dermis. A localised primary infection at the site of entry (chancre or ulcer) is followed by a disseminated secondary stage, then a period of latency, which corresponds with the generation of a vigorous immune response to the organism. Years later, complications of the cardiovascular, neurological and musculoskeletal system occur in approximately one-third of patients.

Two concepts are important when considering the potential impact of condoms in preventing transmission of syphilis. First, infectivity is related to organism load; thus, transmission is more likely during early rather than late disease. Second, primary and secondary lesions, which are likely to be the source of much of the transmitted organisms, may occur in anatomical sites that may not be covered by condoms.

Few studies have addressed the role of condoms in prevention of transmission of syphilis. One case control study from the United States evaluated the association of condom usage with the acquisition of early syphilis in inner city STD clinic attendees.[30] On multivariate analysis, condom usage in the last 3 months was independently associated with a 70 per cent decrease in the risk of early syphilis. A similar result was obtained from a Peruvian study of female sex workers. Consistent condom use in the preceding year was independently associated with a 70 per cent reduction in risk of current syphilis (arbitrarily defined) and a 60 per cent reduction in risk of current or past syphilis.[15]

A number of studies have assessed condom usage in relation to prevalence of positive syphilis serology and yielded mixed results. Uribe-Salas et al. 1996 did not demonstrate any difference in the prevalence of positive serology related to condom usage.[31] A study of syphilis serology in transvestite prostitutes in Italy did not detect a significant difference in rates of TPHA positive tests in "always" versus "inconsistent" condom users, but of 18 individuals who reported consistent condom use in the past 12 months, none was positive for SPHA-IgM (a marker of recently acquired syphilis) as compared to 7 of 53 inconsistent condom users.[32] By contrast, a large study of patterns of sexually transmitted diseases in female sex workers in Indonesia showed that women who reported any condom usage in the last week were significantly less likely to have positive syphilis serology than women who reported no condom usage.[19] Data from these studies may be difficult to interpret as infection may have occurred years before the time period when condom usage was assessed.

Finally, indirect evidence for a protective role for condoms in prevention of syphilis comes from condom intervention programmes in which the prevalence of syphilis declines during the intervention. Roumeliotou et al. in 1988 reported a reduction in prevalence of syphilis from 17.1 to 3.2 per cent in 350 Greek female sex workers over a 3-year intervention period.[18] Similarly, in a group of 824 female sex workers in Japan, prevalence of syphilis fell from 7.5 to 0.5 per cent in a 3-year period which saw a significant rise in consistent condom usage from 6.3 to 25.3 per cent of women.[28]

Tropical STIs and genital ulcer disease

There are three bacterial infections that are often referred to as the tropical STIs. All three are associated with genital ulcers. The commonest infection found in most tropical areas is

69

Chancroid, a painful destructive infection caused by *Haemophilus ducreyi*. The second infection is Lymphogranuloma venereum, which is caused by *Chlamydia trachomatis*, serotypes L1–3, and characterised by transient genital ulceration and long-term blockage of lymphatics resulting in inginual lymphadenopathy and sometimes elephantiasis of the genitalia or legs. The final infection is Donovanosis (also called Granuloma inginale) caused by a bacterium *Calymmatobacterium granulomatis*. This is a rare infection confined to Papua New Guinea, far north Australia, and a few isolated parts of southern Africa. It is characterised by destructive genital ulceration.

There are no published studies that have looked at the protective efficacy of condoms for the prevention of these individual infections. However, studies have been done to demonstrate the usefulness of condoms for the prevention of genital ulcer disease (GUD). A study of female CSWs in Nairobi showed a direct association of GUD and reported condom use. Sixteen per cent of patients presenting with GUD always used condoms, compared with 31 per cent in those who used condoms mostly, 33 per cent in those who used them sometimes, and 45 per cent in those who never used condoms ($p < 0.02$ for trend).[33]

Viral infections

Human immunodeficiency virus (HIV)

Human immunodeficiency virus is a retroviral infection, which causes progressive impairment and destruction of the immune system over a period of years. This eventually renders the individual susceptible to a variety of opportunistic infections, which can affect many organ systems and may ultimately cause death of the infected individual. HIV is transmitted by exchange of body fluids and sexual transmission accounts for the vast majority of infections worldwide.

The absence of vaccine or cure and the inaccessibility of antiretroviral drugs to the majority of infected individuals have sparked great interest in the role of condoms in preventing sexual transmission of HIV. Evidence from laboratory studies suggests that latex condoms do provide a barrier to HIV transmission[34] depsite fears that the presence of small holes may allow virus to penetrate through the latex.[35]

It is believed that breaches of mucosal integrity, such as traumatic micro-abrasions, which may occur during sexual intercourse, or concurrent genital ulceration may facilitate HIV transmission.[3,36] At the individual level, gender and disease stage of the HIV infected partner, coexistent genital infection, and the type of sexual practice may all influence the risk of transmission and may impact on estimates of condom effectiveness.

Studies broadly fall into four categories: prospective studies of seroconversion rates in serodiscordant couples (where one partner is HIV-positive and the other HIV-negative); meta-analyses of such studies; models of transmission dynamics; and indirect evidence from comparisons of prevalence and incidence of HIV in condom users and non-users in a variety of populations.

An early meta-analysis included 11 studies of sexually active, HIV serodiscodant, heterosexual couples.[37] The analysis suggested that condoms were 60–70 per cent effective in preventing HIV transmission. This meant that condom users were 60–70 per cent less likely to acquire HIV as a result of sex with an infected partner than non-condom users. However, this study did not separate data on consistent and inconsistent condom users. Thus, any protective effect would be diluted by episodes of unprotected intercourse included in the inconsistent users group[38] and that the true effectiveness could be considerably higher. In addition, the analysis may have been limited further, as male-to-female and female-to-male transmission were considered together.[39]

Latterly, these issues were addressed in a meta-analysis that included only those studies in which condom usage was stratified into consistent and inconsistent use.[39] The overall effectiveness of consistent condom use in prevention of HIV transmission was found to be at least 90–95 per cent, considerably higher than the earlier estimate (Table 5.2).[37]

Pinkerton and Abramson then used the pooled data from the meta-analysis in a mathematical model, the Bernoulli Process Model, in which each act of sexual intercourse was considered as a separate trial, to derive an absolute estimate of condom effectiveness.[39] Condoms were found to decrease the per-contact probability of male-to-female HIV transmission by 95 per cent. This meant that inconsistent condom users were 20 times more likely to seroconvert following repeated contacts with an HIV-positive partner than consistent users.

Recent case control studies in heterosexual and homosexual/

Table 5.2 Condom use and seropositivity rates in heterosexual serodiscordant couples

Study	Year	Direction of transmission	Condom use	
			Consistent	Inconsistent
Fischl et al.[40,a]	1987	M → F (patients with AIDS)	1/10	12/14
Goedert et al.[41]	1987	M → F (haemophiliacs)	0/6	4/18
Roumelioutou-Karayannis et al.[42,a]	1988	M → F	0/37	12/16
Van der Ende et al.[43,a]	1988	M → F	0/2	0/11
Johnson et al.[44]	1989	M → F	0/4	15/74
Laurian et al.[45,a]	1989	M → F (haemophiliacs)	0/14	3/17
European Study Group[46,a]	1992	M → F	0/16	82/388
Allen et al.[47,a]	1992	M → F	0/4	6/26
Saracco et al.[48,a]	1993	M → F	3/171	6/134
Gumaráes et al.[49]	1995	M → F	7/31	85/173
Allen et al.[47]	1992	F → M	0/5	2/18
European Study Group[46]	1992	F → M	0/8	19/151
Nicolosi et al.[50]	1994	F → M	2/69	12/155
De Vincenzi[51]	1994	M → F and F → M	0/124	12/121
Nicolosi et al.[52]	1994	M → F and F → M	8/96	169/457
Deschamps et al.[53]	1996	M → F and F → M	1/42	19/135
Hira et al.[54]	1997	M → F and F → M	2.3/100 couple years	10.7/100 couple years

Source: based on Pinkerton and Abramson, 1997.[39]
[a] Studies included in Pinkerton and Abramson meta-analysis (1997).
M → F = male-to-female transmission, F → M = female-to-male transmission.

bisexual populations reported a variable reduction in risk of HIV acquisition in condom users. Taneepanichskul *et al.* reported in 1997 a 70 per cent reduction in risk of HIV in condom-using Thai female sex workers.[55] Williams *et al.* in a study of homo/bisexual men in London, described in 1996 odds ratios for HIV of 7.9 (95 per cent CI 2.2–28.9) and 16.2 (95 per cent CI 3.0–86.0) in inconsistent and non-condom users, respectively, as compared with consistent users.[56] Data from a nested case control study of a subgroup of homosexual men in the Chicago MACS cohort suggested that consistent condom usage for receptive anal sex was associated with a significantly lower but notable (15 per cent) seroconversion rate than unprotected receptive anal sex (51 per cent).[57] A study of heterosexual, homo/bisexual men and women STD clinic attendees in Northern Italy reported that regular condom use decreased the risk of HIV infection by 50 per cent compared with no or occasional condom users.[58] However, comparisons between studies are difficult as condom usage was not stratified in a standardised way and the study populations were varied.

A small number of studies have either failed to demonstrate a protective effect for condoms in reduction of HIV transmission[59] or have even shown an increased rate of HIV transmission in condom users.[60] The former study stratified condom use into "ever" and "never" used condoms, and it is likely that very infrequent users would dilute any protective effect. Mnyika *et al.* suggested that condom use was in fact a marker of high-risk behaviour in this population of Tanzanian women.

Finally, results from intervention programmes, which include condom promotion as part of the intervention strategy, indirectly support a protective role for condoms.[61,62]

In summary, consistently and correctly used condoms appear to be highly effective in reducing but not totally eliminating sexual HIV transmission.

Herpes simplex virus (HSV)

Genital herpes is a viral infection resulting in recurrent genital blistering and ulceration. It is caused by Herpes simplex viruses types one and two. HSV-2 is transmitted by genital to genital contact and HSV-1 from mouth to genital contact. The infection can be asymptomatic and infectious virus can be shed from intact skin from any part of the genital tract and surrounding areas or the mucus membranes of the genital tract or mouth.

Laboratory plunger tests have shown that the intact latex condom is impervious to HSV-2.[63] However, as virus can be shed from intact skin which condoms may not cover, they are likely to be less effective for the prevention of herpes than for gonorrhoea or chlamydia. There is only one published study that was specifically designed to determine the efficacy of condoms for HSV prevention. The study was conducted in Costa Rica among 766 women aged 25–59, randomly selected for a national household survey. Of women whose partners had used condoms for 2 years or more 28.9 per cent (SE ± 8.7) were HSV-2 seropositive compared with 33.5 per cent (SE ± 7.8) of those whose partners had used condoms for 1–24 months and 44.3 per cent (SE ± 4.9) in those whose partners had never used condoms.[64] By contrast, a study from Peru in female commercial sex workers showed that consistent condom use was not associated with a lower HSV-2 seroprevalence[15] and a study from Denmark amongst inner city female STD clinic attendees suggested that despite an increase in the proportion of condom users from 6 to 22 per cent between 1984 and 1988 the incidence of genital herpes remained virtually unchanged.[65]

Human papillomavirus (HPV) and associated conditions

There are a large number of HPVs. However, only a minority of these is transmitted sexually. Their association with genital tract tumours into high risk, intermediate risk and low risk further classifies the sexually transmitted HPVs. The low and intermediate risk types usually cause genital warts.

Genital warts can occur anywhere on the genital mucosa or surrounding skin and consequently it is unlikely that condoms will offer complete protection. A case control study from an STD clinic in Sydney showed that males who never used condoms were more than one and a half times more likely to have warts than those who did (OR 1.62 95 per cent CI 1.05–2.52). Men who always used condoms had less than half the likelihood of developing warts than those who did not (OR 0.47 95 per cent CI 0.32–0.72). There was also a significant benefit for women whose partners used condoms ($p = 0.04$).[66] Condoms also appear to improve the clearance rate in males with warts (presumably by reducing re-infection).[67] Finally a case control study in women with flat warts on the cervix showed that these were more common on women whose partners did not use condoms (16 per cent) compared with those who did (12 per cent), $p < 0.05$.[68]

A case control study of 225 married women with squamous cell carcinoma of the cervix and their husbands showed that the husband's failure to use condoms with female CSWs was associated with an increased risk of squamous carcinoma of the cervix. Comparing cases and controls the relative risk for those never or rarely using condoms was 2.05 (95 per cent CI 1.12–3.87).[69] A Danish case control study showed that monogamous women whose partners had ever used condoms were less likely to have carcinoma *in situ* or invasive cervical cancer than who had never used condoms (relative risk 0.2 95 per cent CI 0.1–0.6).[70] However, not all studies have confirmed these findings.[71–74]

Hepatitis A, B and C

Hepatitis A is transmitted via faeco-oral contamination and condoms are unlikely to have any impact on transmission. Hepatitis B (HBV) is transmitted via blood (usually through needle sharing or contamination) and sexually via exchange of body fluids. Latex condoms are impervious to HBV,[75] however there are no published studies to determine whether this has any impact on transmission.

Hepatitis C (HCV) is most commonly transmitted via blood, although sexual transmission does occasionally occur. A study looking at risk factors for HCV acquisition in heterosexual couples did not show any protective efficacy for condoms.[76] However, the study was small and only a minority of couples used condoms.

Human T cell lymphotropic virus type 1 (HLTV 1)

HTLV1 is a retroviral infection that can be transmitted sexually. It is associated with a variety of clinical syndromes including adult T cell leukaemia/lymphoma and tropical spastic paraparesis. Condoms used for more than 50 per cent of sexual encounters over a 3-year period significantly reduce the risk of HLTV 1 infection (OR 0.34 95 per cent CI 0.13–0.89).[77]

Protozoal infections

Trichomonas

Trichomonas vaginalis is a flagellate protozoan, which may present with vaginitis and vaginal discharge of varying severity in women, and occasionally urethritis in men. It is thought to be asymptomatic in 10 to 50 per cent of women and may be present only transiently in men. Infection is confined to the lower genital tract.

The association between condom usage and transmission of *T. vaginalis* has not been extensively studied. However where data exist, condoms appear to have a protective role. A large Taiwanese study of almost 16 000 women in which trichomonas was diagnosed on pap smear samples, reported that condom usage was associated with a 60 per cent reduction in risk of trichomonas.[78]

A number of other studies have demonstrated a protective effect for condoms. Rosenberg *et al.* reported in 1992 a 30 per cent reduction in risk of trichomonas in condom-using women compared with non-condom users.[14] A study of risk factors for genital infection in female sex workers in Amsterdam detected a relative risk for trichomonas of 1.7 (95 per cent CI 1.4–2.1) and 1.8 (95 per cent CI 1.3–2.4) for women who mainly or seldom used condoms for vaginal sex with clients as compared with women who always used condoms.[20] Two further studies reported that absence of condoms or inconsistent use was associated with a greater risk of trichomoniasis.[19,79]

Miscellaneous conditions

Pelvic inflammatory disease (PID) and tubal infertility

Ascending infection of the female genital tract with chlamydia and/or gonorrhoea may result in infection and possible damage to the Fallopian tubes and surrounding tissues. This is termed PID. This in turn, may lead to chronic pelvic pain, infertility and ectopic pregnancies. A case control study of 306 women with PID showed that condom users had a decreased risk of PID when compared with those not using any contraception (relative risk 0.6 95 per cent CI 0.4–0.9).[80]

Condoms, particularly if used over many years, appear to reduce the risk of tubal infertility. Cramer *et al.* studied 283 nulliparous women with tubal infertility and 3883 women admitted for delivery of a live-born child. Women who had ever used barrier contraception were significantly less likely to have tubal infertility than those who had not (relative risk 0.7 95 per cent CI 0.5–0.9). Further analysis of these data revealed that condoms alone were not associated with a significant reduction in tubal infertility whereas when condoms were used together with a spermicide they were (relative risk 0.4 95 per cent CI 0.2–0.9).[81] A smaller case control study confirmed these findings but only when condoms were used for more than 1 year and when the women had sexual intercourse with more than 1 partner (relative risk 0.38 95 per cent CI 0.13–1.00).[82]

Vaginal bacterial flora (anaerobic vaginosis)

The health of the vagina is maintained by bacterial flora, in particular lactobacilli producing hydrogen peroxide. Upset in the balance of bacterial flora may result in an overgrowth with anaerobic bacteria, resulting in a condition called anaerobic vaginosis. A study of 30 women in Finland found that women who were using oral contraceptives and intrauterine devices were at increased risk of anaerobic infection. Whereas those using barrier contraceptives (condoms or diaphragms) were more likely to have maintained the normal vaginal flora.[83]

Estimates of the protective efficacy of condoms for all the STIs and related conditions is summarised in Table 5.3.

Summary

Condoms are highly effective method of preventing many sexually transmitted infections, in particular gonorrhoea, chlamydia, HIV and hepatitis B. They also offer some protection against those infections transmitted, mainly via skin-to-skin contact, in particular human papillomavirus infection and warts. The degree of protection is also dependent upon the user. Couples who use condoms throughout every act of sexual contact will have a high degree of protection.

Table 5.3 Estimated protection offered by latex condoms for various STIs and related conditions

Infection or condition	Estimated protection from condoms	Comments	References
STIs in general	300–50% higher incidence in non or inconsistent users	Cohort study	2
Gonorrhoea	Males: 30–60% reduction for condom users 30–200% higher incidence in non users; Females: 30–60% reduction for condom users	Several cross-sectional and case control studies	8, 11, 12, 13
Chlamydia	Males: 30% reduction for condom users; Females: 40% higher incidence in non or inconsistent users	Several cross-sectional and case control studies; most evidence is in females	11, 20, 26, 27
Urethritis (not due to gonorrhoea or chlamydia)	40% reduction for condom users	Single case control study	11
Syphilis	40–80% reduction for condom users	Several case control and observational studies	15, 18, 30
Genital ulcer disease	65% reduction in consistent condom users	Single cross-sectional study	33
HIV	60–95% reduction for condom users	See text and table 3	
Genital herpes	33% reduction in women whose partners had used condoms for at least 2 years	Single cross-sectional study using type specific HSV serology	64
Human papilloma virus	Males: 62% higher prevalence in condom users 53% reduction for condom users Females: 25% reduction	Two case control studies	66, 68

Table 5.3 (continued)

Infection or condition	Estimated protection from condoms	Comments	References
Cervical cancer	80% reduction for condom users	One case control and one observational study	69, 70
	200% increased risk for non users		
Hepatitis A	No evidence		
Hepatitis B	No evidence		
Hepatitis C	No evidence		
HLTV-1	60% reduction for condom users	Retrospective observational study	77
Trichomonas	70–80% higher incidence in non or inconsistent users	Several case control and observational studies	14, 20, 78
	30–60% reduction in condom users		
PID	40% reduction for long-term condom users	Single case control study	80
Tubal infertility	30% reduction for users of barrier contraception	Two case control studies	81, 82
Anaerobic vaginosis	30–40% higher prevalence in IUD and oral contraceptive users	Single observational study	83
Mycoplasma	60% reduction in consistent users	Single observational study	29

References

1 Judson FN, Ehret JM, Bodin GF, Levin MJ, Rietmeijer CAM. In vitro evaluations of condoms with and without nonoxynol-9 as physical and chemical barriers against Chlamydia trachomatis, Herpes simplex virus type 2, and human immunodeficiency virus. *Sex Trans Dis* 1989; **16**: 51–6.
2 Celentano DD, Nelson KE, Suprasert S *et al*. Epidemiologic risk factors for incident sexually transmitted diseases in young Thai men. *Sex Trans Dis* 1996; **23**: 198–205.
3 Joffe GP, Foxman B, Schmidt AJ, *et al*. Multiple Partners and Partner Choice as Risk Factors for Sexually Transmitted Disease Among Female College Students. *Sex Trans Dis* 1992; **19**: 272–8.
4 Zenilman JM, Weisman CS, Rompalo AM, *et al*. Condom Use to Prevent Incident STIs: The validty of Self-Reported Condom Use. *Sex Trans Dis* 1995; **22**: 15–21.
5 Weir SS, Feldblum PJ. Condom use to prevent incident STIs. (Letter to the Editor.) *Sex Trans Dis* 1994; **23**: 76–7.
6 Galavotti C, Cabral C, Beeker C. (Letter to the Editor.) *Sex Trans Dis* 1996; **23**: 77–9.
7 Kretzschmar M, van Duynhoven THP, Severijnen AJ. Modeling prevention strategies for gonorrhoea and chlamydia using stochastic network simulations. *Am J Epidemiol* 1996; **144**: 306–17.
8 Barlow D. The condom and gonorrhoea. *Lancet* 1977; October 15: 811–13.
9 Hooper RR, Reynolds GH, Jones OG, *et al*. Cohort study of venereal disease. I: The risk of gonorrhoea transmission from infected women to men. *Am J Epidemiol* 1978; **108**: 136–44.
10 Cates W, Holmes KK. Condom efficacy against gonorrhea and non-gonococcal urethritis. *Am J Epidemiol* 1996; **143**: 843–4.
11 Schwartz MA, Lafferty WE, Hughes JP, Handsfield HH. Risk factors for urethritis in heterosexual men. *Sex Trans Dis* 1997; **24**: 449–55.
12 Upchurch DM, Brady WE, Reichart CA, Hook EW III. Behavioral contributions to acquisition of gonorrhea in patients attending an inner city sexually transmitted disease clinic. *J Infect Dis* 1990; **161**: 938–41.
13 Ellen JM, Langer LM, Zimmerman RS, Cabral RJ, Fichtner R. The link between the use of crack cocaine and the sexually transmitted diseases of a clinic population: a comparison of adolescents with adults. *Sex Trans Dis* 1996; **23**: 511–16.
14 Rosenberg MJ, Davidson AJ, Chen J-H, Judson FN, Douglas JM. Barrier contraceptives and sexually transmitted diseases in women: a comparison of female-dependent methods and condoms. *Am J Public Health* 1992; **82**: 669–74.
15 Sànchez J, Gotuzzo E, Escamilla J, *et al*. Gender differences in sexual practices and sexually transmitted infections among adults in Lima, Peru. *Am J Public Health* 1996; **86**: 1098–107.
16 O'Connor CC, Berry G, Rohrsheim R, Donovan B. Sexual health and use of condoms among local and international sex workers in Sydney. *Genitourin Med* 1996; **72**: 47–51.
17 Swaddiwudipong W, Chaovakiratipong C, Siri S, Lerdukanavonge P. Sociodemographic characteristics and incidence of gonorrhoea in prostitutes working near the Thai–Burmese border. *Southeast Asia J Trop Med Public Health*. 1990; **21**: 45–52.
18 Romeliotou A, Papautsakis G, Kallinikos G, Papaevangelou G. Effectiveness of condom use in preventing HIV infection in prostitutes. *Lancet* 1998; **2** (8622): 1249.
19 Joesoef MF, Linnan M, Barrakbah Y, Idajadi A, Kambodji A, Schulz K.

Patterns of sexually transmitted diseases in female sex workers in Surabaya, Indonesia. *In J STD AIDS* 1997; **8:** 576–80.

20 Fennema JSA, van Ameijden EJC, Coutinho RA, van den Hoek A. Clinical sexually transmitted diseases among human immunodeficiency virus-infected and noninfected drug-using prostitutes. *Sex Trans Dis* 1997; **24:** 363–71.

21 Evans BA, Kell PD, Bond RA, MacRae KD. Heterosexual relationships and condom-use in the spread of sexually transmitted diseases to women. *Genitourin Med* 1995; **71:** 291–4.

22 Quinn RW, O'Reilly KR. Contraceptive practices of women attending the sexually transmitted disease clinic in Nashville, Tennessee. *Sex Trans Dis* 1985; **12:** 99–102.

23 Berger GS, Keith L, Moss W. Prevalence of gonorrhoea among women using various methods of contraception. *Brit J Vener Dis* 1975; **51:** 307–9.

24 Keith L, Berer GS, Moss W. Cervical gonorrhea in women using different methods of contraception. *J Am Ven Dis Assoc* 1976; **3:** 17–19.

25 Austin H, Louv WC, Alexander WJ. A case control study of spermicides and gonorrhea. *JAMA* 1984; **251:** 2822–4.

26 Gaydos CA, Howell MR, Pare B *et al. Chlamydia trachomatis* infections in female military recruits. *N Engl J Med* 1998; **339:** 739–44.

27 Ramstedt K, Forssman L, Giesecke J, Granath F. Risk factors for *Chlamydia trachomatis* infection in 6810 young women attending family planning clinics. *Int J STD AIDS* 1992; **3:** 117–22.

28 Tanaka M, Nakayama H, Sakumoto M, Matsumoto T, Akazawa KJ, Kumazawa J. Trends in sexually transmitted diseases and condom use patterns among commercial sex workers in Fumkuoka City, Japan 1990–93. *Genitourin Med,* 1996; **72:** 358–61.

29 McCormack WM, Lee Y-H, Zinner SH. Sexual experience and urethral colonization with genital mycoplasmas. *Ann Intern Med* 1973; **78:** 696–8.

30 Finelli L, Budd J, Spitalny KC. Early syphilis: relationship to sex, drugs and changes in high-risk behavior from 1987–90. *Sex Trans Dis,* 1993; **20:** 90–5.

31 Uribe-Salas F, Del Rio-Chiriboga C, Conde-Glez CJ, *et al.* Prevalence incidence, and determinants of syphilis in female commercial sex workers in Mexico City. *Sex Trans Dis,* 1996; **23:** 121–6.

32 Gattari P, Speziale D, Grillo R *et al.* Syphilis serology among transvestite prostitutes attending an HIV unit in Rome, Italy. *Eur J Epidemiol* 1994; **10:** 683–6

33 Cameron DW, Ngugi EN, Ronald AR *et al.* Condom use prevents genital ulcers in women working as prostitutes. *Sex Trans Dis* 1991; **18:** 188–91.

34 Centres for Disease Control and Prevention. Condoms for the prevention of sexually transmitted diseases. *Morbid Mortal Weekly Rep* 1998; **37:** 133–7.

35 Lytle CD, Routson LB, Seaborn GB, Dixon LG, Bushar HF, Cyr WH. An in vitro evaluation of condoms as barriers to a small virus. *Sex Trans Dis,* 1997; **24:** 161–4.

36 O'Brien TR, Shaffer N, Jaffe HW. Acquisition and transmission of HIV. In: *The medical management of AIDS.* Sande MA, Volberding PA. (eds). Philadelphia: Saunders, 1992; 3–17.

37 Weller SC. A meta-analysis of condom effectiveness in reducing sexually transmitted HIV. *Soc Sci Med* 1993; **36:** 1635–44.

38 Warner DL, Hatcher RA. A meta-analysis of condom effectiveness in reducing sexually transmitted HIV. *Soc Sci Med* 1994; **38:** 1169–70.

39 Pinkerton SD, Abramson PR. Effectiveness of condoms in preventing HIV transmission. *Soc Sci Med* 1997; **44:** 1303–12.

40 Fischl MA, Dickinson GM, Scott GB, Klimas N, Fletcher MA, Parks W. Evaluation of heterosexual partners, children, and household contacts of adults with AIDS. *JAMA* 1997; **257:** 640–4.

41 Goedert JJ, Eyster ME, Biggar RJ, Blattner WA. Heterosexual transmission of

human immunodeficiency virus: association with severe depletion of T-helper lymphocytes in men with hemophilia. *AIDS Res Human Retroviruses* 1987; **3**: 355–61.

42 Romel Roumelioutou-Karayannis A, Nestoridou KA, Mandalaki T, Stefanou T, Papaevangelou G. Heterosexual transmission of HIV in Greece. *AIDS Res Human Retroviruses* 1988; **4**: 233–5.

43 Van der Ende ME, Rothbarth P, Stibbe J. Heterosexual transmission of HIV by haemophiliacs. *BMJ* 1988; **297**: 1102–3.

44 Johnson AM, Pethrick A, Davidson SJ *et al*. Transmission of human immuno-deficiency virus to sexual partners of haemophiliacs. *AIDS* 1989; **3**: 367–72.

45 Laurian Y, Peynet J, Verroust. HIV infection in sexual partners of HIV-seropositive patients with hemophilia. *New Engl J Med* 199; **320**: 183.

46 European Study Group on Heterosexual Transmission of HIV. Comparison of female to male and male to female transmission of HIV in 563 stable couples. *BMJ* 1992; **304**: 809–12.

47 Allen S, Tice J, van de Perre P *et al*. Effect of serotesting with counselling on condom use and seroconversion among HIV discordant couples in Africa. *BMJ* 1992; **304**: 1605–9.

48 Saracco A, Musicco M, Nicolosi A, *et al*. Man-to-woman sexual transmission of HIV: Longitudinal study of 343 steady partners of infected men. *J Acquir Immune Def Syndr* 1993; **6**: 497–502.

49 Guimarães MDC, Muñoz A, Boschi-Pinto C, Castilho EA. For the Rio de Janeiro Heterosexual Study Group. HIV infection among female partners of seropositive men in Brazil. *Am J Epidemiol* 1995; **142**: 538–46.

50 Nicolosi A, Leite MLC, Musicco M, Arici C, Gavazzeni G, Lazzarin A. For the Italian Study Group on HIV heterosexual transmission. The efficiency of male-to-female and female-to-male sexual transmission of the human immuno-deficiency virus: a study of 730 stable couples. *Epidemiology*, 1994; **5**: 750–75.

51 de Vincenzi I. For the European Study Group on Heterosexual Transmission of HIV. A longitudinal study of human immunodeficiency virus transmission by heterosexual partners. *N Engl J Med*, 1994; **331**: 341–6.

52 Nicolosi A, Musicco M, Saracco A, Lazzarin A. For the Italian Study Group on HIV Heterosexual Transmission. Risk factors for woman-to-man sexual transmission of the human immunodeficiency virus. *J Acquir Immun Def Syndr* 1994; **7**: 296–300.

53 Deschamps M-M, Pape JW, Hafner A, Johnson Jr. WD. Heterosexual trans-mission of HIV in Haiti. *Ann Int Med* 1996; **125**: 324–30.

54 Hira SK, Feldblum PJ, Kamanga J, Mukelabai G, Weir SS, Thomas JC. Condom and nonoxynol-9 use and the incidence of HIV infection in serodis-cordant couples in Zambia. *Int J STD AIDS* 1997; **8**: 243–50.

55 Taneepanichskul S, Phuapradit W, Chaturachinda K. Association of contra-ceptives and HIV-1 infection in Thai female commercial sex workers. *Austral New Zealand J Obstet Gynaecol* 1997; **37**: 86–8.

56 Williams DI, Stephenson JM, Hart GJ, Copas A, Johnson AM, Williams IG. A case control study of HIV seroconversion in gay men, 1988–1993: what are the current risk factors? *Genitourin Med*, 1996; **72**: 193–6.

57 Difranceisco W, Ostrow DG, Chmiel JS. Sexual adventurism, high-risk beha-vior, and human immunodeficiency virus-1 seroconversion among the Chicago MACS-CCS Cohort, 1984 to 1992. A case-control study. *Sex Trans Dis*, 1996; 453–60.

58 Parazzini F, D'Oro LC, Nalda L, *et al*. Number of sexual partners, condom use and risk of human immunodeficiency virus infection. *Int J Epidemiol* 1995; **24**: 1197–203.

59 Gomez MP, Bain RM, Major C, Gray H, Read SE. Characteristics of HIV-infected pregnant women in the Bahamas. *J Acquir Immune Def Syndr Hum Retrovirol* 1996; **12**: 400–405.

60 Mnyika KS, Klepp KL, Kvåle G, Ole-King'ori N. Risk factors for HIV-1 Infection among women in the Arusha region of Tanzania. *J Acquir Immun Def Syndr Hum Retrovirol* 1996; **11**: 484–91.

61 Ngugi EN, Plummer FA, Simonsen JN *et al*. Prevention of transmission of human immunodeficiency virus in Africa: Effectiveness of condom promotion and health education among prostitutes. *Lancet* 1988: **2** (8616); 887–90.

62 Laga M, Alary M, Nzila N *et al*. Condom promotion, sexually transmitted diseases treatment, and declining incidence of HIV-1 infection in female Zairian sex workers. *Lancet* 1994; **344** (8917): 246–8.

63 Conant MA, Spicer DW, Smith CD. Herpes simplex virus transmission: condom studies. *Sex Trans Dis* 1983; **11**: 94–5.

64 Oberle MW, Rosero-Bixby L, Lee FK, Sanchez-Braverman M, Nahmias AJ, Guinan ME. Herpes simplex virus type 2 antibodies: high prevalence in monogamous women in Costa Rica. *Am J Trop Med Hyg* 1989; **41**: 224–9.

65 Olivarius F de F, Worm AM, Petersen CS, Kroon S, Lynge E. Sexual behaviour of women attending an inner-city STD clinic before and after a general campaign for safer sex in Denmark. *Genitourin Med* 1992; **68**: 296–9.

66 Wen LM, Estcourt C, Simpson J, Mindel A. Risk factors for the acquisition of genital warts: are condoms protective? *Sex Transm Inf* 1999 (in press).

67 Hippeläinen MI, Hippeläain M, Saarikoski S, Syrjänen K. Clinical course and prognostic factors of human papillomavirus infections on men. *Sex Trans Dis* 1994; **21**: 272–9.

68 Syrjänen K, Väyrynen M, Castrén O, *et al*. Sexual behaviour of women with human papillomavirus (HPV) lesions of the uterine cervix. *Br J Vener Dis* 1984; **60**: 243–8.

69 Thomas DB, Ray RM, Pardthaisong T, *et al*. Prostitution, condom use, and invasive squamous cell cervical cancer in Thailand. *Am J Epidemiol* 1996; **143**: 779–86.

70 Kjaer SK, de Villiers E-M, Dahl C, *et al*. Case-control study of risk factors for cervical neoplasia in Denmark 1: role of the "male factor" in women with one lifetime sexual partner. *Int J Cancer* 1991; **48**: 39–44.

71 Hildesheim A, Brinton LA, Mallin K, *et al*. Barrier and spermicidal contraceptive methods and risk of invasive cervical cancer. *Epidemiology* 1990; **1**: 266–72.

72 Slattery ML, Overall JC, Abbott TM, French TK, Robinson LM, Gardner J. Sexual activity, contraception, genital infections, and cervical cancer: support for a sexually transmitted disease hypothesis. *Am J Epidemiol* 1989; **130**: 248–58.

73 Kreiss JK, Kiviat NB, Plummer FA, *et al*. Human immunodeficiency virus, human papillomavirus, and cervical intraepithelial neoplasia in Nairobi prostitutes. *Sex Trans Dis* 1992; **19**: 54–9.

74 Donnan SPB, Wong FWS, Ho SC, Lau EM, Takashi K, Esteve J. Reproductive and sexual risk factors and human papilloma virus infection in cervical cancer among Hong Kong Chinese. *Int J Epidemiol* 1989; **18**: 32–6.

75 Minuyk GY, Bohme CE, Bowen TJ, *et al*. Efficacy of commercial condoms in the prevention of hepatitis B virus infection. *Gastroenterology* 1987; **93**: 710–14.

76 Osmond DH, Padian NS, Sheppard HW, Glass S, Shiboski SC, Reingold A. Risk factors for hepatitis C virus seropositivity in heterosexual couples. *JAMA* 1993; **269**: 361–5.

77 Gotuzzo E, Sánchez J, Escamilla J, *et al*. Human T cell lymphotropic virus type 1 infection among female sex workers in Peru. *J Infect Dis* 1994; **169**: 754–9.

78 Wang PD, Lin RS. Epidemiologic differences between candidal and trichomonal infections as detected in cytologic smears in Taiwan. *Public Health*, 1995; **109**: 443–450.

79 Morrison CS, Sunkutu MR, Musaba E, Glover LH. Sexually transmitted

disease among married Zambian women: the role of male and female sexual behaviour in prevention and management. *Genitourin Med*, 1997; **73**: 555–7.
80 Kelaghan J, Rubin GL, Ory HW, Layde PM. Barrier-method contraceptives and pelvic inflammatory disease. *JAMA* 1982; **248**: 184–7.
81 Cramer DW, Goldman MB, Schiff I *et al*. The relationship of tubal infertility to barrier method and oral contraceptive use. *JAMA* 1987; **257**: 2446–50.
82 Li De-K, Daling JR, Stergachis AS, Chu J, Weiss NS. Prior condom use and the risk of tubal pregnancy. *Am J Public Health* 1990; **80**: 964–6.
83 Haukkamaa M, Stranden P, Jousimies-Somer H, Siitonen A. Bacterial flora of the cervix in women using different methods of contraception. *Am J Obstet Gynecol* 1986; **154**: 520–4.

6 Spermicides and virucides

D J JEFFRIES, R J AITKEN

The design of new contraceptive methods for the new millennium will have to incorporate a response to the mounting risk of sexually transmitted disease (STD). In the past decade there has been a dramatic global increase in STIs, such that we are currently seeing around 333 million new cases every year. The viral causes of STIs (human immunodeficiency virus [HIV], human papillomaviruses, hepatitis B virus, and herpes simplex viruses) are a particular source of concern because their spread has been so rapid, the pathologies they generate are severe and they do not yield to the antibiotics that are normally used to treat bacterial and protozoal STD. Highly prevalent non-viral diseases such as gonorrhoea and chlamydia are also important however, not just because of the morbidity they induce but because of epidemiological synergy that exists between viral and non-viral forms of STD, such that the latter increase the risk of HIV transmission by three to five fold.[1] Thus it would be advantageous if spermicides of the future should not only target spermatozoa but also the wide range of pathogenic organisms responsible for the world wide spread of STIs.

This objective cannot be achieved with a broad spectrum antibiotic because the vagina possesses a natural bacterial flora that appears to be essential for the preservation of a balanced ecosystem within the vaginal lumen. The low pH and hydrogen peroxide produced by the endogenous Lactobacilli are thought to be particularly important in this respect. Destruction of these organisms, with nonoxynol-9 (N-9) for example, leads to an increased risk of both genital and urinary tract infections.[2,3]

Thus, specificity of action will clearly be an important requirement for any candidate spermicide/microbicide developed for contraceptive use. The feasibility of developing appropriate reagents will, in turn, depend upon our fundamental knowledge of the molecular mechanisms that drive both spermatozoa and the pathogenic entities we wish to target.

Spermicides

The nature of spermicides

Spermicides are generally defined as compounds that are capable of immobilising all the spermatozoa in an ejaculate within 20 seconds.[4] Since the average human ejaculate will contain around 150 million motile spermatozoa, spermicides are inherently toxic compounds that must diffuse rapidly through the aqueous seminal environment to achieve their pharmacological objective. The history of spermicides dates back to van Leewenhoek's eighteenth century discovery that dilution of canine semen with rain-water immobilises dog spermatozoa. By the nineteenth century a variety of miscellaneous spermicidal treatments had been described including electric shock, poisonous heavy metals, beef broth, milk, urine, and a concoction known as "the wife's friend" comprising a cocoa butter suppository impregnated with quinine compounds.[5,6] During the twentieth century a variety of well defined spermicidal agents was discovered that could be classified according to their mechanism of action as (1) enzyme inhibitors such as α-chlorohydrin, (2) substances that attack sulphydryl groups including o-iodosobenzoate, and (3) surface active agents, of which N-9 and sodium dodecyl sulphate are examples in current commercial use.

Surface active agents

For reasons that are not entirely clear, the commercial spermicide industry has decided to focus on N-9 as the reagent of choice and this compound can now be found in a variety of formulations including gels, creams, foams, and films as well as coated on to the surface of medicated condoms. There can be no doubt that N-9 is a powerful surface active agent, immobilising spermatozoa at micromolar concentrations and possibly providing some protection against both HIV (see below) and non-viral STIs including gonorrhoea and chlamydia.[7-9]

Apart from N-9, a variety of other surface active compounds are capable of immobilising spermatozoa with high efficiency including membrane stabilisers such as propranolol, and a range of antibiotics and antiseptic compounds of which the magainins, C31G, parabens, and chlorhexidine are recent examples.[10–12] All of these compounds are effective spermicides and several of them have been shown to exhibit anti-HIV activity *in vitro*.[10–13] However, like N-9, they all lack specificity in terms of their mechanism of action. As a consequence, these reagents are likely to attack the native vaginal microflora and the tissues of the female reproductive tract in addition to their intended targets, with adverse consequences.[2]

Oxidative stress

Spermatozoa are extremely susceptible to oxidative stress by virtue of their high polyunsaturated acid content and diminished capacity for antioxidant defence.[4] Somatic cells are generally protected from oxidative attack through the action of powerful antioxidant enzymes (catalase, glutathione peroxidase, and superoxide dismutase) that reside in the cytoplasmic space. However, spermatozoa discharge most of their cytoplasm immediately before spermiation, and what cytoplasmic space does exist is concentrated in the midpiece of the cell. The plasma membrane overlying the sperm tail is therefore particularly susceptible to oxidative stress with the result that oxidising agents such as hydrogen (or lipid) peroxide are powerful inhibitors of sperm motility.[14–17] Recently, a series of spermicidal organometallic complexes containing vanadium (IV) have been synthesised which also appear to act through the induction of free radical generation and oxidative stress, inducing changes in the spermatozoa (annexin V binding and DNA fragmentation) that resemble apoptosis.[18]

The induction of oxidative stress through the topical administration of pro-oxidant compounds certainly has much to commend it, as an approach to contraception. The tissues and bacterial flora of the lower female reproductive tract are adapted to cope with oxidants such as hydrogen peroxide, because the latter is generated by the vaginal Lactobacilli that protect against infection.[19] On the other hand, high concentrations of hydrogen peroxide are known to disrupt the infectivity of reproductive pathogens including chlamydia, HIV, and herpes simplex.[19–21]

As a consequence of these factors, peroxide-based spermicides should be able to exhibit a selective destructive action on spermatozoa and pathogenic micro-organisms in the vagina, without compromising the normal cellular or microbiological integrity of the female reproductive tract.

Despite the promise offered by pro-oxidant spermicides, the fact that reagents such as hydrogen peroxide and metallocene vanadium complexes induce DNA fragmentation in the spermatozoa[18,22] does raise significant concerns about the safety of this approach. Such concern stems from epidemiological studies indicating that the DNA fragmentation and oxidative base damage induced in human spermatozoa by smoking,[23] are associated with a four-fold increased risk of childhood cancer in the offspring.[24] Thus, if a redox-active spermicide were not completely effective and DNA-damaged spermatozoa were to fertilise the oocyte, then there would be a potential risk of serious morbidity in the offspring.

Sulphydryl reactive agents

A related group of potential spermicides comprises reagents that attack sulphydryl groups on mammalian spermatozoa. According to how they act, thiol reactive agents can be subdivided into: oxidising; alkylating; or mercaptide-forming. We have already discussed the potential use of oxidising agents such as hydrogen peroxide in a contraceptive context and there are commercial products on the market that feature this reagent as the active principle. Cysteamine is another recent example of a thiol reactive agent with spermicidal properties.[25] Cysteamine appears to be effective as a topical contraceptive in the rabbit even though the immediate effects on sperm motility are extremely weak. This compound does however have a delayed effect on sperm motility and can also disrupt other aspects of sperm function including the acrosome reaction.[25] The slow loss of sperm motility observed with cysteamine might be due to the formation of mixed disulphides with intracellular glutathione followed by disruption of the glutathione cycle and the resultant induction of peroxidative damage to the sperm plasma membrane. The latter would then be expected to disrupt the fertilising potential of the spermatozoa without the need for a complete suppression of sperm motility.[14] Membrane permeant thiols, such as 2-mercaptoethanol, will also disrupt the fertilising potential of human spermatozoa without affecting motility, by inhibiting the tyrosine phosphorylation events associated with capacitation; a process that is critically important for the creation of a functional spermatozoon.[26] As indicated below, the mechanism of action of such compounds may hold the key to the future development of effective, specific spermicides/microbicides free from harmful side effects.

Future prospects

To date spermicide research has focused on the development of reagents that completely immobilise human spermatozoa within 20 seconds. The result of this strategy has been the identification of highly active molecules such as N-9 that are certainly effective contraceptives but operate via mechanisms that are devoid of subtlety or specificity. As a result, this compound exhibits a broad spectrum of cytotoxic effects attacking not just spermatozoa but also the tissues and microbial populations of the lower female reproductive tract, generating unwanted side effects that can be serious. The future of spermicide development must lie in the realisation that sperm function can be disrupted by interfering with any one of the myriad cellular events leading up to the process of fertilisation without, necessarily, suppressing sperm motility. A comprehensive review of sperm cell biology is beyond the scope of this review but Figure 6.1 illustrates some of the key features of fertilisation and the range of compounds that are known to interfere with specific events. Vulnerable processes include (1) the development of hyperactivated motility, a specific form of movement that is essential for penetration of the egg investments and may be driven by nitric oxide, (2) capacitation, a maturation event completed during the migration of spermatozoa through the female reproductive tract and involving a redox-regulated induction of tyrosine phosphorylation, (3) the acrosome reaction, a secretory event that takes place on the surface of the egg following sperm-egg recognition and (4) sperm-oocyte fusion.

A possible clue to the development of spermicides with anti-HIV activity may lie in the fact that both sperm–egg interaction and the association of an enveloped virus with its host cell are united by their common dependence upon an act of membrane fusion. Any reagent that interferes with the fusogenicity of a spermatozoon should also interfere with the infectivity of an enveloped virus. Moreover, there are reasons to believe that both of these processes share a similar underlying biochemistry.[28]

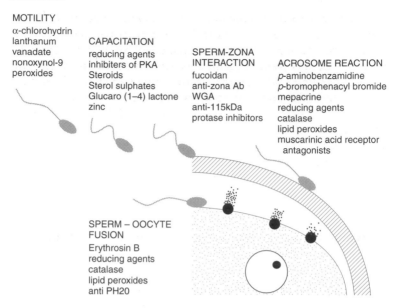

MOTILITY
α-chlorohydrin
lanthanum
vanadate
nonoxynol-9
peroxides

CAPACITATION
reducing agents
inhibiters of PKA
Steroids
Sterol sulphates
Glucaro (1–4) lactone
zinc

SPERM-ZONA
INTERACTION
fucoidan
anti-zona Ab
WGA
anti-115kDa
protase inhibitors

ACROSOME REACTION
p-aminobenzamidine
p-bromophenacyl bromide
mepacrine
reducing agents
catalase
lipid peroxides
muscarinic acid receptor
antagonists

SPERM – OOCYTE
FUSION
Erythrosin B
reducing agents
catalase
lipid peroxides
anti PH20

Figure 6.1   Examples of reagents that have been shown to disrupt various components of the fertilisation process.

In this light it is not surprising that the membrane-perturbing properties of N-9 confer upon this compound both spermicidal and virucidal properties. Similarly, the dependence of membrane fusion on membrane fluidity renders both fertilisation and HIV infectivity susceptible to oxidants that attack the unsaturated fatty acids involved in conferring this property upon biological membranes. The apparent dependence of viral fusion and fertilisation on sulphydryl groups also renders both of these processes susceptible to thiol reactive compounds such as cysteamine.[25] Such observations represent a promising beginning to the development of safe effective spermicides with anti-STD activity. Further possibilities for the development of reagents capable of controlling the fertilising potential of human spermatozoa and impeding the infectivity of reproductive pathogens such as HIV are certain to arise as our understanding of the underlying biochemistry improves.

Virucides

Despite evidence that nonoxynol-9 (N-9) inactivates certain sexually transmitted pathogens *in vitro*, including HIV,[29–33] *Neisseria gonorrhoeae*,[34] *Chlamydia trachomatis*,[35,36] *Haemophilus ducreyi*,[37] *Treponema pallidum*,[38] *Trichomonas vaginalis*,[34] and herpes simplex virus,[39,40] there is no conclusive evidence that this spermicide, or any other preparation used intra-vaginally, will assist in preventing infection *in vivo*. Indeed, concerns over mucosal damage and alteration of the normal vaginal flora raise concerns that N-9 and other currently available spermicides may, in fact, increase the risk of infection with HIV and other STD agents. Until potent and less toxic compounds can be developed for use as vaginal virucides/microbicides, condoms remain the only effective means of preventing sexually transmitted infection and no effective chemical agents can be recommended for this purpose.

Clinical studies of putative vaginal virucides/microbicides

Clinical studies of N-9 used as a virucide/microbicide have produced conflicting results. Early studies were of limited value for a number of reasons, which included differences in study designs, compliance problems, small sample sizes, and questions about the validity of self-reported data. A randomised controlled trial of a commercial contraceptive sponge containing 1000 mg of N-9 was conducted in 138 female commercial sex workers in Nairobi, Kenya.[41] This study was stopped early because of an increase in HIV infection among the users of the sponge (rate ratio 1.6, 95 per cent CI 0.8–2.8) and the frequency of genital ulceration and vulvitis was greater in the N-9 group when compared with that in the placebo group. There are, however, several features about this study that make interpretation difficult. First, the amount of N-9 administered was high when compared to the amount in other spermicidal preparations. Second, the placebo used was not a sponge but a vaginal cream; thus it is impossible to determine whether the sponge itself contributed to the pathological findings. Third, the women were using the sponge 14 times per week on average: it is possible that less frequent use would have been less damaging to the genital tract. Finally, as only self-reported data were collected, the compliance level is open to question. Despite the lack of effect on HIV transmission, Kreiss *et al.* reported a decrease in cervical gonorrhoea in the treated group.[41]

In a cohort study in female prostitutes in Cameroon, Zekeng *et al.* reported a lower rate of HIV infection among women who consistently used N-9 suppositories (100 mg N-9) than among

91

those who used them less consistently (rate ratio 0.1, 95 per cent CI 0.1–0.6).[42] In a study of 110 Zambian couples in whom only the male was HIV positive, a rate ratio of 0.5 (95 per cent CI 0.1–3.8) was recorded among women who reported 100 per cent use of N-9 as compared to those who reported less frequent use.[43] However, the size and design of the Cameroon and Zambian studies limit the significance that can be attached to these results.

Other studies have focused more on the potential toxicity of surfactants used intravaginally. In a phase I study of intra-vaginal N-9 conducted in Thailand, a preparation containing 150 mg was administered 6 hourly for 14 days.[44] Damage to the vaginal epithelium was observed in 43 per cent of the women and the lesions resolved within 7 days of stopping the treatment. In a larger study, 343 women were randomised to receive either 72 mg of N-9, or placebo, at rates of use up to 22 vaginal insertions per week. The use of N-9 was associated with a slightly higher rate of vaginal irritation but with no obvious ulceration.[45]

In a dose-ranging study of N-9 conducted in the Dominican Republic, participants were randomised to receive N-9 suppositories (150 mg N-9) at rates of one suppository every other day, or once, twice or four times per day, for a two week period.[46] There were 35 women in each group and a further group of women received placebo suppositories (four times daily for two weeks). The rates of reported symptoms (vaginal itching and burning) were similar in the N-9 and placebo groups. However, colposcopic examination revealed epithelial disruption of the vagina and cervix which increased in parallel with the rate of N-9 application. While the degree of epithelial disruption in those who applied the N-9 suppositories every other day was comparable to that in the placebo group, the frequency of epithelial damage was 2.5 and 5 times higher in those who used the suppositories once or twice and four times daily, respectively.

Recently, the results of a double-blind, placebo-controlled study of N-9 film (70 mg N-9) or placebo film, conducted in 1292 HIV-negative female commercial sex workers in Cameroon, have been reported.[47] The film was inserted into the vagina before intercourse and all of the women were issued with latex condoms and were instructed to ask their partners to use them. At monthly visits, the women were examined colposcopically, and endocervical specimens were tested for *Neisseria gonorrhoeae* and *Chlamydia trachomatis* with DNA probes. Blood samples were taken and tested for HIV antibody on each visit. The rates of HIV infection were 6.7 cases per 100 women-years in the N-9 group and 6.6 cases per 10 women-years in the placebo group (rate ratio 1.0, 95 per cent CI 0.7–1.5). The rates of genital lesions were 42.2 and 33.5 (cases per 100 women-years) respectively (rate ratio 1.3, 95 per cent CI 1.0–1.6).

Gonorrhoea occurred at rates of 33.3 cases per 100 women-years in the N-9 group and 31.1 in the placebo group (rate ratio 1.1, 95 per cent CI 0.8–1.4) and the corresponding rates for chlamydia were 20.6 and 22.2 cases per 100 women-years (rate ratio 0.9, 95 per cent CI 0.7–1.3). The women reported that condoms were used for 90 per cent of the sexual acts. Thus, in this well-conducted study, the use of N-9 vaginal film did not reduce the rate of new HIV, gonorrhoea, or chlamydial infection in this group of female prostitutes who used condoms and, in addition, received treatment for STIs as they were diagnosed.

The rate of condom use was higher than had been anticipated but the fact that HIV seroconversion occurred in 94 women means that the study had a power of at least 90 per cent to detect a 50 per cent reduction in HIV infection with N-9. However, although on questioning the women were able to explain how to use the N-9 film correctly, there is no evidence to indicate that this delivery system has been tested to ensure that it provides reliable and consistent coating of the genital tract mucosa.

There is one report of a safety study of a different surfactant spermicide, menfegol.[48] One hundred and twenty-five women were randomised to receive menfegol foaming tablets or placebo tablets at different frequencies of vaginal insertion. The rate of cervical and vaginal lesions was high in both groups and the rate of lesion formation increased with the frequency of application.

Future Prospects

In addition to the possibility, as indicated previously, that new strategies for developing spermicidal compounds may also lead to the discovery of new virucides/microbicides, several compounds are undergoing assessment in early clinical trials. These include gramicidin, a peptide antibiotic, which has been used as a spermicide and shown selectively to inhibit HIV in cell culture,[49] dextrin-2-sulphate, a sulphated polyanionic compound, and Procept-2000, a naphthalene sulphonate polymer.[51] The low toxicity profile of sulphated polyanions and other polymers may render them more acceptable for topical use in the sensitive ecosystem of the female genital tract. The likelihood that their effect on HIV is virustatic, rather than virucidal, however, brings into question their suitability for use as single agents. It may be necessary to combine them with a low dose of an agent such as N-9, which is known to destroy the infectivity of HIV and other STD agents.

Conclusion

Spermicides with proven efficacy and acceptably low toxicity have been available for many years. There are prospects for the development of new strategies for spermicidal activity which will allow higher specificity. At present, no spermicidal compounds or any other agent can be used as a virucide/microbicide to prevent transmission of HIV or other STD agents. The mucosal damage and change in the normal flora demonstrated with N-9, is likely to occur with all available surfactant spermicides and these effects are likely to enhance the risks of acquiring infection.

References

1 Stone KM. HIV, other STIs and barriers. In: Mauck CM, Cordero M, Gabilnick HL, Spieler JM, Rivera R, eds. *Barrier contraceptives: current status and future prospects.* New York 1994.
2 Ngugi E, Kreiss J, Holmes K *et al.* Efficacy of nonoxynol-9 contraceptive sponge use in preventing heterosexual acquisition of HIV in Nairobi prostitutes. In: Mauck CM, Cordero M, Gabilnick HL, Spieler JM, Rivera R, eds. *Barrier contraceptives: current status and future prospects.* New York 1994.
3 Fihn SD, Boyko EJ, Normand EH, Chen CL, Grafton JR, Hunt M. Association between use of spermicide-coated condoms and Escherichia-coli urinary tract infection in your women. *Am J Epidemiol* 1996; **144**: 512–20.
4 Sander FV, Cramer SD. A practical approach for testing the spermicidal action of chemical contraceptives. *Hum Fertil* 1941; **6**: 134–7.
5 Jefferson WL. Non-ionic surfactant spermicidal agents. *Brit J Fam Plann* 1986; **11**: 131–5.
6 Mann T, Lutwak-Mann C. *Male reproductive function and semen.* New York: Springer-Verlag, 1981.
7 Chijoke PC, Zaman S, Pearson RM. Comparison of the potency of d-propranolol, chlorhexidine, and nonoxynol-9 in the Sander-Cramer test. *Contraception* 1986; **34**: 207–11.
8 Cook RL, Rosenberg MJ. Do spermicides containing nonoxynol-9 prevent sexually transmitted infections? A meta-analysis. *Sex Trans Dis* 1998; **25**: 144–50.
9 Wittkowski KM, Susser E, Dietz K. The protective effect of condoms and nonoxynol-9 against HIV infection. *Am J Public Health* 1998; **88**: 590–6.
10 Thompson KA, Malamud D, Storey BT. Assessment of the anti-microbial agent C31G as a spermicide: comparison with nonoxynol-9. *Contraception* 1996; **53**: 313–8.
11 Edelstein MC, Gretz GE, Bauer TJ, Fulgham DL, Alexander NJ, Archer DF.

Studies on the in vitro spermicidal activity of synthetic magainins. *Fertil Steril* 1991; **55**: 647–9.

12 Song B-L, Li H-Y, Peng D-R. In vitro spermicidal activity of parabens against human spermatozoa. *Contraception* 1989; **39**: 331–5.

13 Harrison C, Chantler E. The effect of nonoxynol-9 and chlorhexidine on HIV and sperm in vitro. *Int J STD AIDS* 1998; **9**: 92–7.

14 Aitken RJ, Fisher H. Reactive oxygen species generation and human spermatozoa: the balance of benefit and risk. *Bioessays* 1994; **16**: 259–267.

15 Aitken RJ, Buckingham D, Harkiss D. Use of a xanthine oxidase oxidant generating system to investigate the cytotoxic effects of reactive oxygen species on human spermatozoa. *J Reprod Fertil* 1992; **97**: 441–50.

16 Jones R, Mann T, Sherins RJ. Peroxidative breakdown of phospholipids in human spermatozoa: spermicidal effects of fatty acid peroxides and protective action of seminal plasma. *Fertil Steril* 1979; **31**: 531–7.

17 Jones R, Mann T, Sherins RJ. Adverse effects of peroxidized lipid on human spermatozoa. *Proc R Soc Lond B* 1978; **201**: 413–7.

18 D'Cruz JD, Ghosh P, Uckun FM. Spermicidal activity of metallocene complexes containing vanadium (V) in humans. *Biol Reprod* 1998; **58**: 1515–26.

19 Hillier SL, Krohn MA, Klebanoff SJ, Eschenbach DA. The relationship of hydrogen peroxide-producing lactobacilli to bacterial vaginosis and genital microflora in pregnant women. *Obstet Gynececol* 1992; **79**: 369–73.

20 Roberts C, Antonoplos P. Inactivation of human immunodeficiency virus type 1, hepatitis A virus, respiratory syncytial virus, vaccinia virus, herpes simplex virus type 1, and poliovirus type 2 by hydrogen peroxide gas plasma sterilization. *Am J Infect Cont* 1998; **26**: 94–101.

21 Ranjbar S, Holmes H. Influence of hydrogen peroxide on the infectivity of human immunodeficiency virus. *Free Rad Biol Med* 1996, **20**. 573–7.

22 Hughes CM, Lewis SEM, McKelvey-Martin VJ, Thompson W. A comparison of baseline and induced DNA damage in human spermatozoa from fertile and infertile men using a modified comet assay. *Mol Hum Reprod* 1996; **2**: 613–20.

23 Fraga CG, Motchnik PA, Wyrobek AJ, Rempel DM, Ames BN. Smoking and low antioxidant levels increase oxidative damage to sperm DNA. *Mut Res* 1996; **351**: 199–203.

24 Ji BT, Shu XO, Linet MS, Zheng W, Wacholder S, Gao YT, Ying DM, Jin F. Paternal cigarette smoking and the risk of childhood cancer among offspring of nonsmoking mothers. *J Natl Cancer Inst* 1997; **89**: 238–44.

25 Anderson RA, Feathergill K, Kirkpatrick R *et al*. Characterization of cysteamine as a potential contraceptive anti-HIV agent. *J Androl* 1998; **18**: 37–49.

26 Aitken RJ, M Paterson M, Fisher H, Buckingham DW, van Duin M. Redox regulation of tyrosine phosphorylation in human spermatozoa is involved in the control of human sperm function. *J Cell Sci* 1995; **108**: 2017–25.

27 Ryser HJ-P, Levy EM, Mandel R, Disciullo GJ. Inhibition of human immunodeficiency virus infection by agents that interfere with thioldisulphide interchange upon virus-receptor interaction. *Proc Nat Acad Sci USA* 1994; **91**: 4559–63.

28 Blobel CP, Wolfsberg TG, Turck CW, Myles DG, Primakoff P, White JM. A potential fusion peptide and an integrin ligand domain in a protein active in sperm–egg fusion. *Nature* 1992; **356**: 248–52.

29 Hicks DR, Martin LS, Getchell JP, *et al*. Inactivation of HTLV-III/LAV-infected cultures of normal human lymphocytes by nonoxynol-9 in vitro. *Lancet* 1985; **2**: 1422–3.

30 Polsky B, Baron PA, Gold JWM, Smith JL, Jensen RH, Armstrong D. In-vitro inactivation of HIV-1 by contraceptive sponge containing nonoxynol-9. *Lancet* 1988; **1**: 1456.

31 Malkowsky M, Newell A, Dalgleish AG. Inactivation of HIV by nonoxynol-9. *Lancet* 1988; **1**: 645.
32 Rietmeijer CAM, Krebs JW, Feorino PM, Judson FN. Condoms as physical and chemical barriers against human immunodeficiency virus. *JAMA* 1988; **259**: 1851–3.
33 O'Connor TJ, Kinchington D, Kangro HO, Jeffries DJ. The activity of candidate virucidal agents, low pH, and genital secretions against HIV-1 *in vitro*. *Int J STD and AIDS* 1995; **6**: 267–72.
34 Bolch OH Jr, Warren JC. In-vitro effects of Emko on *Neisseria gonorrhoeae* and *Trichomonas vaginalis*. *Am J Obstet Gynecol* 1973; **115**: 1145–8.
35 Benes S, McCormack WM. Inhibition of growth of *Chlamydia trachomatis* by nonoxynol-9 in vitro. *Antimicrob Agent Chemother* 1985; **27**: 724–6.
36 Kelly JP, Reynolds RB, Stagno S, Louv WC, Alexander WJ. In-vitro activity of the spermicide nonoxynol-9 against *Chlamydia trachomatis*. *Antimicrob Agent Chemother* 1985; **27**: 760–2.
37 Jones BM, Geary I, Lee ME, Duerden BI. Susceptibility of *Haemophilus ducreyi* to spermicidal compounds *in vitro*. *Genitourin Med* 1991; **67**: 268–9.
38 Singh B, Cutler JC, Utidjian HMD. Studies on the development of a vaginal preparation providing both prophylaxis against venereal disease and other genital infections and contraception. II Effect *in vitro* of vaginal contraceptive and non-contraceptive preparations on *Treponema pallidum* and *Neisseria gonorrhoeae*. *Br J Vener Dis* 1972; **48**: 57–64.
39 Singh B, Posti B, Cutler JC. Virucidal effect of certain chemical contraceptives on type 2 herpesvirus. *Am J Obstet Gynecol* 1976; **126**: 422–5.
40 Asculai SS, Weis MT, Rancourt MW, Kupferberg AB. Inactivation of herpes simplex viruses by nonionic surfactants. *Antimicrob Agent Chemother* 1978; **13**: 686–90.
41 Kreiss J, Ngugi E, Holmes KK, *et al.* Efficacy of nonoxynol-9 contraceptive sponge use in preventing heterosexual acquisition of HIV in Nairobi protitutes. *JAMA* 1992; **268**: 477–82.
42 Zekeng L, Feldblum PJ, Oliver RM, Kaptue L. Barrier contraceptive use and HIV infection among high-risk women in Cameroon. *AIDS* 1993; **7**: 725–31.
43 Hira SK, Feldblum PJ, Kamanga J, Mukelabai G, Weir SS, Thomas JC. Condom and nonoxynol-9 use and the incidence of HIV infection in sero-discordant couples in Zambia. *Int J STD AIDS* 1997; **8**: 243–50.
44 Niruthisard S, Roddy RE, Chutivongse S. The effects of frequent nonoxynol-9 use on the vaginal and cervical mucosa. *Sex Transm Dis* 1991; **18**: 176–9.
45 Niruthisard S, Roddy RE, Chutivongse S. Use of nonoxynol-9 and reduction in rate of gonococcal and chlamydial cervical infections. *Lancet* 1992; **339**: 1371–5.
46 Roddy RE, Cordero M, Cordero C, Fortney JA. A dosing study of nonoxynol-9 and genital irritation. *Int J STD AIDS* 1993; **4**: 165–70.
47 Roddy RE, Zekeng L, Ryan KA, *et al.* A controlled trial of nonoxynol-9 film to reduce male-to-female transmission of sexually transmitted diseases. *New Eng J Med* 1998; **339**: 504–10.
48 Goeman J, Ndoye I, Sakho LM, *et al.* Frequent use of menfegol spermicidal vaginal foaming tablets associated with a high incidence of genital lesions. *J Infec Dis* 1995; **171**: 1611–4.
49 Bourinbaiar S, Lee Huang S. Comparative in-vitro study of contraceptive agents with anti-HIV activity: gramicidin, nonoxynol-9 and gossypol. *Contraception* 1994; **49**: 131–7.
50 Javan CM, Gooderham NJ, Edwards RJ, *et al.* Anti HIV type 1 activity of sulfated derivatives of dextrin against primary isolates of HIV type 1 in lymphocytes and monocyte-derived macrophages. *AIDS Res Hum Retro* 1997; **13**: 875–80.
51 Rusconi S, Moonis M, Merrell DP. Naphthalene sulphonate polymers with CD4 blocking and anti-human immunodeficiency virus type 1 activity. *Antimicrob Agent Chemother* 1996; **40**: 234–6.

7 Use of condoms: data from population surveys

ANNE C GRUNSEIT, ANNE M JOHNSON

Introduction

In this chapter, we examine data from population surveys which measure the pattern of use of condoms in different parts of the world, examine variability in use over time, and discuss the demographic and behavioural factors that may influence use. The role and effectiveness of condoms in preventing pregnancy and STIs are reviewed in Chapters 4 and 5.

The conclusions that we are able to draw are necessarily broad because of the differences between surveys in the type of population sampled, and the questions asked. Sample and question design depend on the purpose of the survey. Prior to the HIV epidemic, general population surveys focused on use of condoms for contraception. Trends in use over time have been influenced by new technologies such as the oral contraceptive pill. Since the emergence of the AIDS epidemic, public health campaigns have placed emphasis on the use of condoms for HIV and STD prevention. Thus the specific measures of condom use in large population-based surveys are influenced by the research focus and the sociocultural context of different studies.

Methodological issues

We have tried to draw primarily on surveys undertaken in random population samples. However, sampling frames vary between countries and over time. For example, surveys in the 1970s largely restricted their questions to married women at a time when it was thought inappropriate to ask single women about contraceptive use. There have been major changes in sexual behaviour over the last 30 years, characterised by earlier age of first intercourse, increasing numbers of sexual partners, and general acceptance of sex before marriage as a social norm.[1] Therefore, contemporary surveys have not only sampled broader populations, but also recent reports may reflect increased willingness to acknowledge contraceptive practice that comes with a more tolerant social context.

Condom use over the last 30 years has been influenced by two important factors. On the one hand, the emergence of new, more reliable methods of contraception (oral contraception, IUCD and surgical sterilisation) provided competing choices with the condom as a means of contraception. On the other hand, condoms have been increasingly promoted over the last 15 years for prophylaxis not only against pregnancy, but also for protection from HIV and STIs. Thus, it is frequently impossible in large scale surveys to disentangle the use of condoms for contraception and fo the prevention of STIs.

Given these methodological difficulties, it is difficult to define with certainty the factors influencing condom use, such that this chapter is focused largely on descriptions of the available data.

Condom use for contraception in the pre-AIDS era

Table 7.1 shows use of condoms for contraception in a number of developed countries in the 1970s, prior to the advent of HIV/AIDS, at a time when the oral contraceptive pill had been recently introduced. It is unfortunate that these studies only report on married women's contraceptive patterns. McEwan *et al.* remark that asking single women to report on their current contraceptive use may have been considered offensive in the 1970s and therefore data from that time period is incomplete.[2]

There is some variability between the countries listed in Table 7.1 in level of condom use, although this may be due to the different samples generated (for example, those from England and Wales are from "ever married" women and those from Australia are currently married). However, use of condoms does not exceed one-third of the sample in any of these studies (Table 7.1). Note that these studies essentially report *any* use of condoms and therefore there is no information concerning consistency of use.

Table 7.1   Proportion (per cent) of married women of "reproductive age" whose partners use condoms in different countries

Country	Year of survey	Current condom use
Australia[a]	1970/71	9
Belgium	1971	10
Denmark	1970	20
England and Wales[b]	1970	31
Finland	1972	31
France	1972	8
Italy	1976	16
Netherlands	1975	10
Norway	1977	15

Sources: All data apart from those quoted for Australia, and England and Wales, derived from Hubert et al. (1998)[3]; [a] From a study conducted in Melbourne only of main method of contraception for married women aged 15–49 (Siedlecky, 1986)[4]; [b] McEwan et al. (1997).[2]

Condom and contraceptive pill use from the pre-AIDS to AIDS era

Table 7.2 is derived from national surveys undertaken in England and Wales, and Table 7.3 shows data collated by Piccinino and Mosher[5] in a review of contraceptive use among women interviewed in the National Survey of Family Growth in the United States in 1982, 1988, and 1995.

The data from England and Wales (Table 7.2) show a decline in condom use from 1970 to 1975 with a subsequent upturn to 1970 levels by 1990. Increasing contraceptive pill usage is seen throughout the same period. According to the later data shown in Table 7.3, in the United States there has been a steady increase in use of condoms between 1982 and 1995. Further, between 1988 and 1995, there appears to have been a decline in pill usage for those women younger than 39 years. Taking both tables

Table 7.2   Current condom and contraceptive pill use as a percentage of ever married women aged 16–41 years who used any form of contraception in England and Wales

Age	1970		1975		1990/91	
	Condoms	Pill	Condoms	Pill	Condoms	Pill
All ages	31	21	22	36	32	40

Source: data derived from McEwan et al. (1997).[2]

Table 7.3   Condom and contraceptive pill use in last month as a percentage of those women age 15–44 years who used any form of contraception in United States

Age	1982		1988		1995	
	Condoms	Pill	Condoms	Pill	Condoms	Pill
15–19	21	64	33	59	37	44
20–24	11	55	55	68	28	52
25–39	11	35	16	45	24	39
30–34	12	16	12	22	18	28
35–39	12	6	12	5	17	11
40–44	11	1	11	3	12	6
All ages	12	28	15	31	20	27

Source: data derived from Piccinino and Mosher (1998).[5]

together, the decline in condom use in the earlier period may relate to change in contraceptive practice, whereas the movement seen in the later period may reflect changes in HIV/STD prevention. This finds some support when these data are examined by marital status: there is little change from 1988 to 1995 among the *married* group for either method, but increased condom use and decreased pill use for *never married* women.[5] Thus the pattern of change in condom use over the pre-AIDS era through to the advent of HIV/AIDS reflects the tensions between the context of, and the need for, contraception and STD prevention (for further discussion regarding partnership status and condom use see section headed "Condom use and cohabitation status" below).

Unfortunately, in many other recent surveys, it is difficult to distinguish between use of condoms for pregnancy prevention and use for prevention of HIV/STD. In many cases condoms may be used for both purposes. However, trends over the pre-AIDS to AIDS eras would seem to suggest that there has been a resurgence in the popularity of condoms which may reasonably be attributed to the HIV threat.

Condom use in the era of HIV/AIDS

Large scale surveys of condom usage have been part of the process of documenting risk of HIV infection since early in the epidemic. The measures representing condom use, however, have varied markedly between studies. Condom use has been described in terms of: use ever (from once in a lifetime onwards); consistency of usage over a specified time period; use at first occasion of intercourse; and use at most recent intercourse. The diversity of variables collected makes comparisons between surveys difficult. The different measures allow some comparison between countries and within countries over time.

Condom use at first intercourse

Studies from the United States, Australia and Britain all suggest that there has been a recent increase in condom use at first intercourse.[1,4,6,7] Data from the British survey[1] indicate that an increase in condom use at first intercourse can be dated to the mid-1980s (Figure 7.1). In Britain, by 1990, over 60 per cent of men and women reported using a condom at first intercourse. Throughout the two decades before this, condom use at first intercourse was stable despite the increasing popularity of oral contraceptives in the early 1970s, report of possible side-effects of the pill later in that decade, and changing sexual behaviour patterns throughout the period. These data suggest, as proposed above, that the recent upturn in condom use at first intercourse may have resulted from AIDS public education campaigns.

Condom use at first intercourse is also related to age at first intercourse. While direct comparisons between surveys is difficult because of the different timing and age structure of the samples, surveys in the industrialised world consistently show that condom use at first intercourse is least frequent among those whose coitarche is before 16 years of age.[a,1,7,8] There is evidence from the same studies, however, that use of *any* form of contraception increases with increasing age at first intercourse. Thus although the likelihood of use of other methods of contraception also tends to increase when first sexual intercourse occurs after the age of 16 years,[1,8] condom use remains the most popular form of contraception at first intercourse at any age.

Ever use

In terms of the prevention of HIV transmission, use of a condom ever (which theoretically combines those who have

---

[a] Note that the study by Grunseit[7] is not a random based survey. The data are drawn from a national study of trade apprentices attending technical and further education colleges aged 15 to 56.

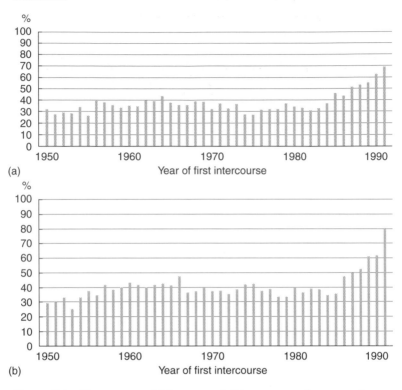

Figure 7.1 Percentage of (a) men and (b) women using a condom at first intercourse by year of first intercourse. Values for 1991 are based on data for 5 months.
Adapted from Johnson et al. (1994).[1]

used a condom once in a lifetime and those who have used them consistently) may at first seem fruitless. However, when looked at across a number of different countries, this measure may be seen as a useful indicator of exposure to condoms at the population level. For example, Cleland and Ferry[9] described in 1995 the results of random sample surveys of individuals aged 15 years or older co-ordinated by the WHO/GPA undertaken in 15 resource-poor nations in 1990.

Table 7.4 shows that there is extremely wide variation in "ever use" of condoms among those with any sexual experience, ranging from 5.9 per cent of women (14.8 per cent of men) in Togo to 84 per cent of women (91 per cent of men) in West Germany. In general, ever use of condoms in industrialised

102

Table 7.4 Proportion (per cent) of sexually experienced people using condoms ever and accessibility by country

Country	Men[b]	Women[b]	Condom access
Belgium[a]	71.0	59.6	na
Burundi	18.5	7.3	37
Central African Republic	21.0	6.8	15
Côte d'Ivoire	30.3	9.3	38
East Germany[a]	75.9	60.7	100[c]
France[a]	69.1	55.5	na
Guinea Bissau	33.0	12.3	17
Kenya	16.4	8.7	na
Lesotho	16.1	8.0	na
Mauritius	50.8	35.8	na
Netherlands[a]	79.5	74.0	na
Portugal[a]	65.8	48.0	na
Singapore	65.8	50.7	na
Sri Lanka	12.2	10.8	na
Switzerland[a]	86.1	80.6	na
Tanzania	14.0	8.5	3.0[c]
Thailand	52.3	21.5	na
Togo	14.8	5.9	21
Britain	80.8	72.0	100[c]
West Germany[a]	91.0	84.0	100[c]

Source: data derived from Mehryar (1995),[10] except for [a] European data from Hubert et al. (1998).[3] [b] Proportion of respondents (18–49 years except Switzerland 18–45 years) who had ever had sex. [c] Condom access as the proportion of adults that had heard of condoms, were aware of a supply source and living and/or working within 30 minutes (60 minutes for Togo) of that source (Mehryar, 1995).[10]
na, data not available.

nations exceeds two-thirds of men, while in developing countries experience of condoms is much less frequent. In each of the African countries surveyed, "ever use" of condoms among men was below one-third of the population.

Descriptive data such as these cannot account for the reasons underlying this variability in use or its impact on STD and HIV transmission. However, from these data it may be said that in countries having the most severe epidemics of HIV and STD, condom use is the least frequent. This serves both to fuel the epidemic and to hinder control strategies where use of condoms is limited to only a minority of the population. Many factors influence the non-use of condoms including availability, cost, cultural acceptability, perceived value, and desire to procreate. These factors are discussed in greater detail in Chapter 11. However, access to condoms is a factor which must be addressed before condom promotion campaigns can achieve any success. Table 7.4 demonstrates that in countries where condom use is limited, access to condoms is similarly limited.

What is also notable about the data in Table 7.4, is the uniformly lower proportions of women reporting condom use compared with men. This is consistent throughout developing,[5] and developed countries,[3] younger cohorts,[11] and general population samples.[1] Assuming that for every heterosexual sexual act involving a condom there would theoretically be one woman and one man reporting that a condom had been used, this discrepancy appears counter-intuitive. However, a number of researchers have sought to explain this discrepancy and in doing so highlight some important issues pertinent to the measurement of condom use by large scale survey.

First, Dubois-Arber and Spencer[12] noted in 1998 this disparity between men's and women's reported rates of condom use in Europe and suggest that it may be an artefact of an over-sampling of high partner-turnover (and therefore high condom-using) men, and/or under-representation of comparable women (for example, sex workers). These authors also hypothesise that given that condoms are a male-controlled prophylactic, women may not consider that *they themselves* have used them. Second, in a more sociocultural vein, Dubois-Arber and Spencer[12] observe that the greater limitations placed on women's sexual autonomy, and the concomitant kudos associated with men's, may also widen the gap in rate at which women and men admit to sexual activity, particularly that which may be construed as occurring outside a committed relationship. As evidence, they noted that those countries which had high levels of condom use overall also had a narrower gap between men and women's usage, perhaps indicating greater acceptance of condoms generally. Further, reporting between the sexes tended to be more comparable in countries where condoms were to be used widely as a contraceptive, as this also improved their acceptability for both women and men.

In understanding the disparity in condom use by men and women, in addition to issues of error due to social acceptability, it is important to consider the impact of sampling strategies on reported use. Surveys sample individuals not partnerships. As we discuss below, condom use varies by age and partnership type. Since women tend to form sexual partnerships with men older than themselves,[13-16] women will be systematically reporting the behaviour of men older than themselves. Older men, in turn, tend to have lower rates of condom use than younger men. Thus women's lower rates for age of reporting may, in part, be a function of the (older) men they are partnered with.

Changes in condom use with age

Describing condom use at last intercourse from large scale surveys by age group affords an interesting profile of the fluctuations that commonly occur throughout an individual's sexual career. As may be seen in Table 7.5, condom use at last intercourse steadily declines with increasing age.

Several factors may be operative in producing such an age effect. First, Shaw (1992)[18] and others suggest that people are primarily interested in preventing pregnancy rather than STIs. Therefore, alternative contraceptive methods such as the pill replace condoms as people become older, more sexually experienced, and enter into established relationships.[19,21–23] For example, Træen, Lewin and Sundet (1992)[24] reported that among their random sample of 1161 sexually active Norwegian 17 to 19-year-olds, 51.4 per cent used condoms at first intercourse and 7 per cent used oral contraception. However, at last intercourse, only 31.4 per cent used condoms and 38 per cent used oral contraception. Second, several researchers have found condom use to decrease with years of sexual experience (as opposed to just age)[14,15,25,26] and with increasing frequency of intercourse.[15,25,27]

Table 7.5 Condom use (percentage) at last intercourse by age (years) in surveys conducted since 1992

Country	18–19	20–24	25–29	30–39	40–49	All ages
Australia[a]	59.9	42.4	27.7	14.0	–	36.0
Finland[b]	50	33.5	25.2	27.9	19.2	28.4
France[b]	41.4	24.7	11.5	10.5	8.5	13.9
Switzerland[b]	53.8	34.1	20.9	18.2	13.9	23.0
	18–24	25–34	35–44	45–59		All ages
Britain[c]	29.9	21.5	17.9	13.0		19.8
United States[c]	31.1	20.1	12.5	4.7		16.8

Sources: [a] Grunseit (1998)[7]; [b] Dubois and Spencer (1998)[12]; [c] Michael et al. (1998).[17]

However, it should be noted that the later coitus is initiated, the more likely a condom will be used at first intercourse.[8,26,28] Third, Johnson et al. report that for Britain, all measures of condom use (ever, in last year, in last 4 weeks, and at last intercourse) showed a decline in prevalence of use with age for both sexes.[1] The greater reported "ever use" of condoms among younger men and women in particular suggests a generational effect towards greater use of condoms in recent generations. This is consistent with the increased use of condoms at first intercourse over time, also observed in a number of studies.[1,29] Thus when looking at the effect of "age" on condom use, the interrelationship of age of initiation, increasing sexual experience with age, and generation have to be taken into account.

Condom use and partnership status

HIV prevention campaigns have promoted the use of condoms, particularly in casual relationships. A number of surveys have examined condom use in relationships to both number and type of partnership. However, very few surveys have collected detailed information on consistency of use in relation to numbers and type of partnership.

Table 7.6 shows data on condom use in the last 12 months by number of partners in the last 12 months for a number of European countries. These show a consistent increase in the use of condoms with increasing numbers of partners. In multivariate analysis in the British survey, multiple partnership remained associated with increased condom use after controlling for age and marital status.[1]

Table 7.6   Condom use (percentage) in the last 12 months by number of partners in the last 12 months

	Netherlands	France	Belgium	Britain	
				Male	Female
1	21.7	27.5	21.2	33.2	24.8
2	49.2	59.8	52.2	55.9	39.6
3–4	66.7	70.1	72.4	61.8	52.3
5+	54.5	77.5	71.9	71.6	60.4

Sources: European data derived from Hubert et al. (1998)[3] and British data derived from Johnson et al. (1994).[1]

Condom use and cohabitation status

The argument presented earlier, that contraception rather than STD prevention is a prime motivator in condom use and is influenced by relationship status, finds resonance in patterns of use over the last 12 months by cohabitation status. The European surveys detailed in Table 7.7 consistently demonstrate that condom use is less prevalent among those who are living with a partner than those who are not (whether or not they are married). A multivariate analysis in the British survey similarly indicates much greater use of condoms by single as compared with married people. Cohabiting respondents used condoms more than single, but less than married respondents. This effect was independent of age and number of partners. These data may reflect the decision of couples in long-term relationships, symbolised by marriage, to adopt a more reliable and permanent method of contraception, in combination with a perceived reduction in the need for protection from STIs.

Further evidence may be found in data from the household Family and Fertility Survey undertaken in France in 1994.[29] Of men who reported using condoms in the last month who were also cohabiting with their partner, 74 per cent said that it was for the purpose of preventing pregnancy and 6 per cent said it was to protect against STIs. The proportions for women were 90 and 6 per cent respectively. For those men not cohabiting with a partner, only 7 per cent reported that condom use in the last month was for contraceptive purposes, 33 per cent for STIs/HIV prevention and 58 per cent said it was for both. The corresponding percentages for cohabiting women were 15, 35, and 49 per cent. Thus use of condoms among cohabiting couples appears

Table 7.7 Condom use (percentage) among those who have had at least one sexual partner in last 12 months by cohabitation status

	Netherlands[a]	France[a]	Belgium[a]	Britain[b]	
				Male	Female
Cohabiting (i.e. married or living with a partner)	20.7	23.4	18.3	28.6	22.7
Not cohabiting	33.3	52.1	17.3	61.0	39.1

Sources: European data derived from Hubert et al. (1998)[3] and British data derived from Johnson et al. (1994).[1]
[a] Of respondents 18–49 years. [b] Of respondents 16–59 years.

to be, in the main, motivated by pregnancy prevention rather than prevention of STIs and/or HIV.

Condom use and casual partnerships

Mathematical models of the HIV epidemic suggest that short-term, casual partnerships may be particularly important in fuelling the HIV epidemic[30] as well as maintaining transmission of other STIs. UNAIDS (1998)[31] have suggested that an indicator of success of HIV prevention programmes may be to monitor the proportion of people using condoms in casual partnerships. While this indicator is available in a number of countries, its interpretation is problematic, since this measure requires: a definition of casual partnership; the use of a comparable denominator between studies; and a comparable measure of the proportion of the population who engage in casual partnerships. We found the currently collated data difficult to interpret, and it has therefore not been presented here. However, from our attempt to synthesise some of the data, it has become evident that a standardised "inventory" of sexual behaviour questions, useful for interpreting trends in behaviours, and allowing comparisons between populations, is urgently required.

Consistency of condom use

In addition to questions of condom use by types of partners, more information is required on consistency of use. De Vincenzi et al. (1993)[32] demonstrated that consistent condom use in stable HIV discordant partners was required to prevent HIV transmission. Inconsistent use is a common cause of both unwanted pregnancy and STD transmission. However, few data are available in this degree of detail from population surveys, and this aspect is therefore not pursued in depth here.

Conclusions

We have presented a brief overview from the extensive literature on condom use from general population surveys. Emphasis has been placed on the methodological difficulties in making temporal and international comparisons caused by the varying sampling strategies and questions asked in different surveys.

The data indicate that condoms have been and continue to be, an important method of contraception. Their popularity waned with the widespread introduction of new, more reliable, contraceptive technologies in the 1970s, but there is some evidence of increasing use since the emergence of the AIDS epidemic. Condom use varies markedly between countries, being less frequent in resource-poor than industrialised countries.

Although condom use has generally increased at first intercourse, condoms are least used among those who have first intercourse before the age of 16, who are less likely to use any form of contraception. Condom use tends to decline with increasing age, and with marriage or cohabitation. Further, there is some evidence from recent surveys that condoms are more likely to be used among those with multiple partners. These associations may be related both to the tendency to use more permanent methods of contraception in long-term relationships as well as a perceived need to protect from STD/HIV in casual relationships, but survey data are generally insufficiently detailed to test these hypotheses.

Population measures of condom use are important in monitoring contraception use and response to STD/HIV prevention campaigns. Such public health surveillance could be achieved more effectively and efficiently by use of standardised questions and comparable sampling frames between populations and over time.

Acknowledgements

We thank Barbara Beaton for clerical assistance and Andrew Copas for statistical data from the British survey.

References

1 Johnson A, Wadsworth J, Wellings K, Field J. *Sexual attitudes and lifestyles.* Oxford: Blackwell Scientific, 1994.

2 McEwan J, Wadsworth J, Johnson AM, Wellings K, Field J. Changes in the use of contraceptive methods in England and Wales over two decades: Margaret Bones's surveys and the National Survey of Sexual Attitudes and Lifestyles. *Br J Fam Plann* 1997; **23**: 5–8.

3 Hubert M, Bajos N, Sandfort T. *Sexual behaviour and HIV/AIDS in Europe.* London: UCL Press, 1998.

4 Siedlecky S. Current usage of and towards contraception in Australia. *Healthright* 1986; **6**: 7–16.

5 Piccinino LJ, Mosher WD. Trends in contraceptive use in the United States: 1982–95. *Fam Plann Perspect* 1998; **30**: 4–10, 46.

6 Mauldon J, Luker K. The effects of contraceptive education on method use at first intercourse. *Fam Plann Perspect* 1996; **26**: 19–24, 41.

7 Grunseit AC. Sex, techs and HIV: gender and HIV response in a national

sample of trade apprentices. Doctoral dissertation, Macquarie University, Sydney, Australia, 1998.

8   Kraft P, Rise J, Træen B. The HIV epidemic and changes in the use of contraception among Norwegian adolescents. *AIDS* 1990; **4**: 673–8.

9   Cleland J, Ferry B. *Sexual behaviour and AIDS in the developing world*. London: Taylor and Francis, 1995.

10 Mehryar A. Condoms: awareness, attitudes and use. In: Cleland J, Ferry B, eds. *Sexual behaviour and AIDS in the developing world*. London: Taylor and Francis, 1995.

11 Svenson L, Carmel S, Varnhagen C. A review of the knowledge, attitudes and behaviours of university students concerning HIV/AIDS. *Health Prom Int* 1997; **12**: 61–8.

12 Dubois-Arber F, Spencer B. Condom use. In: Hubert M, Bajos N, Sandfort T, eds. *Sexual behaviour and HIV/AIDS in Europe*. London: UCL Press, 1998.

13 Bozon M, Kontula O. Sexual initiation and gender in Europe: a cross-cultural analysis of trends in the twentieth century. In: Hubert M, Bajos N, Sandfort T, eds. *Sexual behaviour and HIV/AIDs in Europe*. London: UCL Press, 1998.

14 Lindsay J, Smith A, Rosenthal D. *Secondary students, HIV/AIDS and sexual health 1997*. La Trobe University: Centre for the Study of Sexually Transmissible Diseases, 1997.

15 Træen B, Lewin B, Sundt JM. The real and the ideal; gender differences in heterosexual behaviour among Norwegian adolescents. *J Commun Appl Soc Psychol* 1992; **2**: 227–37.

16 Wadsworth J, Johnson AM, Wellings K, Field J. What's in a mean? An examination of the inconsistency between men and women reporting sexual partnerships. *J R Statist Soc* 196; **159**: 111–23.

17 Michael RT, Wadsworth J, Feinlaub J, Johnson AM, Laumann EO, Wellings K. Private sexual behavior, public opinion, and public health policy related in sexually transmitted diseases: A US-British comparison. *Am J Public Health* 1998; **88**: 749–54.

18 Shaw J. Teenagers and sexually transmitted disease: understanding the barriers to safe behaviour. *Proc Austral Soc Hum Biol* 1992; **5**: 187–200.

19 Dunne M, Donald M, Lucke J, Nilsson R, Ballard R, Raphael B. Age-related increase in sexual behaviours and decrease in regular condom use among adolescents in Australia. *Int J STDs AIDS* 1994; **5**: 41–7.

20 Ingham R, Woodcock A, Stenner K. The limitations of rational decision-making models as applied to young people's sexual behaviour. In: Aggleton P, Davies P, Hart G, eds. *AIDS: rights, risk and reason*. London: The Falmer Press, 1992.

21 Lewis J, Malow R, Ireland S. HIV/AIDS risk in heterosexual college students. *Journal of American College Health* 1997; **45**: 147–58.

22 Pilkington CJ, Kern W, Indest D. Is safer sex necessary with a "safe" partner? Condom use and romantic feelings. *J Sex Res* 1994; **31**: 203–10.

23 Wyn, J. *Young women's health: the challenge of sexually transmitted diseases (Working Paper No. 8)*. Melbourne: Youth Research Centre, Institute of Education, 1993.

24 Træen B, Lewin B, Sundet JM. Use of birth control pills and condoms among 17–19-year-old adolescents in Norway: contraceptive versus protective behaviour? *AIDS Care* 1992; **4**: 371–80.

25 Fergusson D, Lynskey M, Horwood L. AIDS knowledge and condom use in a birth cohort of 16 year olds. *N Z Med J* 1994; **107**: 480–8.

26 Stigum H, Magnus P, Veierod M, Bakketeig L. Impact on sexually transmitted disease spread of increased condom use by young females, 1987–1992. *Int J Epidemiol* 1995; **24**: 813–20.

27 Abraham C, Sheeran P, Abrams D, Spears R. Health beliefs and teenage condom use: a prospective study. *Psychol Health* 1996; **11**: 641–55.

28 Faulkenberry R, Vincent M, James A, Johnson W. Coital behaviors, attitudes, and knowledge of students who experience early coitus. *Adolescence* 1987; **86**: 321–32.
29 Toulemon L, Leridon H. Contraceptive practices and trends in France. *Fam Plann Perspect* 1998; **30**: 114–20.
30 Robinson NJ, Mulder DW, Auvert B, Hayes KJ. Modelling the impact of alternative HIV intervention strategies in rural Uganda. *AIDS* 1995; **9**: 1263–70.
31 UNAIDS/WHO. *Report on the global HIV/AIDS epidemic*. Geneva: Joint United Nations Programme on HIV/AIDS (UNAIDS)/World Health Organziation, 1998.
32 De Vincenzi I, for the European Study Group on Heterosexual Transmission of HIV. A longitudinal study of human immunodeficiency virus transmission by heterosexual partners. *N Engl J Med* 1994; **331**: 341–6.

8 Condoms and commercial sex

ADRIAN MINDEL, CLAUDIA ESTCOURT

The terms "Prostitute", "sex worker", "commercial sex worker", "escort", "call girl", "gigolo", "rent boy", are just a few which have been used to describe individuals who engage in sexual activity with another person, known or unknown, in exchange for material gain or other considerations. Social politics and cultural values may determine the exact nature of the transaction, but the concept of exchange of sexual services for currency, and/or the provision of one or more of the necessities of daily living (food, clothing, protection and possibly drugs)[1] is a common theme worldwide.

In global terms, the largely covert nature of commercial sexual encounters has made reliable estimation of the number of commercial sex workers (CSWs) and the prevalence of commercial sex work almost impossible. However, it does appear that the vast majority of CSWs are poor urban women.[2] In some subcultures, paying for sex is common place. A Thai study of 2417 young military recruits in 1991 reported that 81 per cent gave a history of contact with a female CSW: just over half the sample reported contact in the last year, and 17 per cent in the last month.[3] In the UK national survey of sexual behaviour, 7 per cent of men reported ever having paid for sex.[4]

Recent increases in travel and tourism have opened up the international commercial sex industry. "Sex tourism", typified by men from developed countries travelling to less well developed countries in pursuit of cheap sex, exotic sex, or sex with a particular type of CSW who may be unavailable in their own society, is no longer a novel concept. CSWs may relocate internationally to their target market. Women and men from developing countries have been lured away from their communities by the promise of well paid, respectable work in the cities or even in exciting overseas locations, only to discover that the job amounts to commercial sex work and that they have no means of returning home.

Commercial sex work may contribute to the spread of sexually transmitted infections (STIs) for a variety of reasons. These may vary in significance geographically and over time. Traditionally it is believed that increased numbers of sexual partners and frequent partner change render sex workers vulnerable to infection and potentially more likely to transmit infection than people with fewer partners.[2] In some countries CSWs do have high rates of sexually transmitted infection and HIV, and in some African cities HIV prevalence in female CSWs is over 60 per cent[5] and prevalence of one or more sexually transmitted infections over 75 per cent.[6] However, rates of sexually transmitted infection in CSWs vary enormously across the world and even within subsections of the sex-working population in the same city. In Sydney, rates of sexually transmitted infection in Australian born female CSWs are very low, in sharp contrast to much higher prevalences in international CSWs.[7] It is proposed that a small group of individuals such as this could then act as a core group of transmitters, able to spread infection into the general community.[8]

Other factors may be of greater importance in different situations. Stringent social policies designed to control sex work by criminalisation combined with stigmatising attitudes from the general community have marginalised sex workers and often prevented them from accessing the health care they need. Where health care provision has been made available, it has often been inappropriate or linked to the criminal justice system. Criminalisation of the industry also denies the CSWs health and safety standards, which may decrease their ability to negotiate safer sex with clients.

Outside of paid sex work, evidence for both female and male CSWs suggests that condom usage is low. In addition, it appears that some subgroups of CSWs may have high numbers of non-commercial partners.[9] Both of these factors may contribute to channelling of infection into the general community.

Finally, the role of clients of CSWs in the spread of infection must be considered. The little that is known of this group suggests that sexual risk behaviour extends outside the paid sexual encounter and that rates of sexually transmitted infection are high.[8] Work on male clients of male CSWs suggests that many identify themselves as heterosexual and report non-commercial sex with multiple male and female partners.[8]

Clearly, the role of commercial sex in the spread of sexually transmitted infections is complex and the promotion of condoms within the commercial sex industry is a crucial aspect of all STI control programmes.

Frequency of condom use

The use of condoms within the sex industry as a means of reducing the risk of STIs, particularly for soldiers, was first widely promoted during the first world war. This philosophy was extended during the second world war when allied and German troops were issued with condoms particularly for use with commercial sex workers (see Chapter 1). After the second world war the increasing availability of antibiotics reduced public anxiety about STIs and interest in the use of condoms within the sex industry waned. However, with the advent of the AIDS pandemic in the early 1980s, personal and public health interest in the use of condoms was re-awakened.

Various methods have been used to assess condom use by CSWs and clients in the commercial sex industry. These include: using questions about number of acts protected, with a scale of always to never; calculating the proportion based on protection of the most recent act or the last 5 or 10 acts; using retrospective coital logs, or counting the number of condoms used.[12] Although there is some variation between the methods, at a population level they are broadly comparable.

In the last 15 years numerous studies have been done to determine the proportion of CSWs who use condoms and the factors involved in use and non-use. These studies have revealed that there is a very large variation in condom use around the world. In many developed countries condoms are widely and consistently used by female CSWs for commercial sex[7,13-33] (Table 8.1). However, some female CSWs particularly those who have recently migrated from developing countries have a less consistent pattern of condom use. In Sydney, Australia local CSWs attending an STD clinic used condoms consistently 92 per cent of the time compared with 21 per cent of the international CSWs (mostly Thai and Chinese) (OR 4.5 95 per cent CI 3.1–6.5).[7]

Lower rates of condom use have also been found in many inner

Table 8.1 Condom use by commercial sex workers in developed countries

Place	Date	Number, sex[a] and place of work	Percentage using condoms for commercial sex	Percentage using condoms with regular partners	Comments	Reference
Plovdix, Bulgaria	Not stated	200 streets, hotels, and brothels	74%	3%	Percentage always using condoms	13
Athens, Greece	1985–7	350	66% in 1985, 98% in 1987	NS	Greek CSWs are registered and undergo 3-monthly compulsory health checks	14
Amsterdam	1985–7	117 drug using CSWs	Vaginal sex – 22% always, 74% sometimes, 4% never Oral sex – 23% always, 68% sometimes, 9% never	NS		15
New York, USA	1986–7	78	85% vaginal 86% oral	NS		16
San Francisco, USA	1986–7	181 street	54% always, 40% sometimes, 6% never	5% always, 20% sometimes, 76% never		17
Sydney, Australia	1986–8	231 STD clinic	Vaginal sex – 69% always, 3% never Oral sex – 33% always	Vaginal sex – 12% always, 68% never		18
Amsterdam, Holland	1986–92	108 drug using CSWs	21% in 1986, 33% in 1987, 31% in 1988, 64% in 1989/90 and 58% in 1991/2 always used condoms	NS	Cohort of 108. However, only 26 followed for the full period	19

Table 8.1 (continued)

Place	Date	Number, sex[a] and place of work	Percentage using condoms for commercial sex	Percentage using condoms with regular partners	Comments	Reference
Ghent, Belgium	1988–9	154	Vaginal sex – 61% often, 26% sometimes, 13% never Anal sex – 3% often, 20% sometimes, 77% never	NS		20
9 cities in Italy	1988–92	102	96% always, 4% never	5% always, 32% sometimes, 63% never	Poor condom users were mostly drug users	21
London, England	1989–90	280 STD clinics, streets, and magistrates courts	98% always for vaginal sex, 83% for oral sex, and 50% for anal sex	12% for vaginal, 6% for oral, and 25% for anal sex	Only a small minority admitted to anal sex with clients and non-paying partners	22
Singapore	1990	806 STD clinic	75%	NS		23
9 European cities	1990–1	959 variety of settings	80% always 2% never	82% never	Fewer women who were IDVUs used condoms with clients (73% vs. 82% for non-users)	24
Copenhagen, Denmark	1990–1	327	95% for vaginal sex 98% for oral sex	9–25% for vaginal, 11–25% for oral sex	Subset of European study (above)	25
Fukuoka, Japan	1990–3	79 STD clinic	6–25%	NS		26
Amsterdam, Holland	1991	201 STD clinic and "windows"	66% always, 5% never or seldom	NS		27

Location	Year	Sample			Comments	Ref.
Miami, New York and San Francisco	1991–92	419 men and women	46% vaginal sex 53% anal sex 31% oral sex	23% vaginal sex 17% anal sex 11% oral sex	Crack cocaine users	28
Sydney, Australia	1991–3	91 local CSWs STD clinic	92% consistent use over the last 3 months	54% consistent use over the last 3 months		7
		123 international CSWs STD clinic	21% consistent use over the last 3 months	8% consistent use over the last 3 months		
Singapore	1992	296	75%	NS		29
Melbourne, Australia	1994	321 brothel, escort agency, and street	99% for vaginal and anal sex	40% for vaginal and 45% for anal sex		30
Nevada, USA	1995	44	100%	NS	Condoms are legally required in Nevada's brothels	31

[a] Female unless otherwise stated.
NS, not stated.
IVDU – Intravenous drug user.

city intravenous drug users who are involved in the commercial sex industry.[15,19,21,28] A study from Miami, San Francisco and New York showed that condoms were used consistently less than 50 per cent of the time with paid partners of crack cocaine smokers.[28] Some drug users, who do not identify as commercial sex workers, use sex as a source of income to fund their drug purchases. Condom use in these men and women is low. A study in London found that 59 per cent of heroin using males and 65 per cent of heroin using females rarely or never used condoms for vaginal sex.[32]

In the developing world most studies in the 1980s suggested that condoms were seldom used within the commercial sex industry (Table 8.2).[6,33–59] However, condom promotion campaigns have resulted in a marked increase in condom use in many countries. In Thailand "The 100 per cent Condom Program" has resulted in an increase of condom use from less than 20 per cent before 1989 to over 90 per cent in 1994.[60] Unfortunately, the utilisation of condoms in some developing countries remains poor.[49,52,54,58]

Most studies have only considered vaginal sex. The use of condoms for anal sex (see Chapter 9) and for oral sex within the commercial sex industry has been poorly documented. The few studies that have been done suggest that condoms are used less consistently for these activities than for vaginal sex.[15,18,22,25,28,46,51] For example in Brazil condoms were used with 21–68 per cent of clients for oral sex, 31–81 per cent for anal sex and 51–97 per cent for vaginal sex[46] and in Sydney condoms were used for 69 per cent of vaginal sex compared with 33 per cent for oral sex.[18]

A consistent theme from many of the studies is the observation that female CSWs use condoms far less commonly with non-paying partners (including regular and non-regular partners and pimps) than with paying partners for all types of sexual activity.[7,13,17,18,21,22,24,25,28,30,46,49–51,54,55] As an example, in Brazil, a study of 600 female CSWs revealed that for commercial sex, condoms were used 51–97 per cent for vaginal sex and 31–81 per cent for anal sex, whereas for non-paying partners condoms were used 5–15 per cent for vaginal sex and 5–10 per cent for anal sex.[46] Condoms are considered as "tools of the trade" and consequently used to demarcate private from commercial sexual activity in some settings.[61] With condom use becoming almost universal in most commercial sex, this distinction may become greater. Some women consider that they are so careful at work

Table 8.2 Condom use by commercial sex workers in developing countries

Place	Date	Number, sex[a] and place of work	Percentage using condoms for commercial sex	Percentage using condoms with regular partners	Comments	Reference
Mae Scot district near the Thai-Burmese border	1988	238	89% with <20% of clients 11% with >20% of clients	NS		33
Kinshasa, Zaire	1988	1233, hotel, home and street	6–20% "regular use"	NS		6
Kinshasa, Zaire	1988–91	531 CSWs initially HIV-antibody negative	11% before intervention 52–68% after	NS	Intervention STI management health education and free condoms	34
Jakarta, Indonesia	Not stated	600 male transvestites	50% for receptive anal sex	NS	Safer sex including simulated vaginal sex and masturbation were offered by many	35
Kinshasa, Zaire	1985	377 from bars and hotels	23%	NS		36
Nairobi, Kenya	1985–5	363	1985: 7–10% some; 1986: 3–11% always; 21–44% sometimes, and 19–42% never after health promotion	NS	Health promotion and condom distribution	37
Dakar, Ziguirchor, Kaolack, Senegal	1985–90	1710 STD clinics	10–34% always, 55–79% sometimes, and 5–28% never	NS		38

Table 8.2 (continued)

Place	Date	Number, sex[a] and place of work	Percentage using condoms for commercial sex	Percentage using condoms with regular partners	Comments	Reference
Callao, Peru	1986	140	3%	NS		39
Nairobi, Kenya	1986–7	202	2% always, 73% some or most, 26% never	NS	Condom use increased after health promotion and condom provisions	40
	1987–8	379	7% always, 88% some or most, 5% never			
Accra, Ghana	1987	71 community based	6% always, 36% never	NS	Education intervention by local health workers	41
	1988	148 community based	48% always, 23% never			
	1991	107 community based	64% always, 1% never			
Serekunda, and Farafenni, Gambia	1989–90	121 bars	44–77%	NS	Condom use greater in "high class" bars and for clients who paid more	42
Korogocho, Machakos and Tika, Kenya	1989–90	299 CSWs	4.6% before and 36.5% after intervention	NS	Intervention involved identification, peer education, STI control and condom promotion	43
Chiang Mai, Thailand	1989–94	1174 brothel male CSWs	21–56% never	NS	Higher non-condom use in men who were HIV positive (56%)	44
Khon Kaen City, Thailand	1990–1	217 brothel based	74% increasing to over 93%	NS	Condom use during the previous night. Condom use increased after the	

Location	Year	Sample	Condom use		Comments	Ref
São Paulo, Campinos, Santos, Brazil	1990–91	600 – 200 from each city	51–97% for vaginal 31–81% for anal 21–68% for oral	5–15% for vaginal, 5–10% for anal sex	Women of higher socio-economic status more likely to use condoms for vaginal sex with clients	46
Bulawayo, Zimbabwe	1990–2	705 bars	18% before and 66% after intervention	NS	Intervention involved identification, peer education, STI control, and condom promotion	43
Lima, Peru	1991–2	284 registered 116 unregistered	50% 38%	NS	Condom use over the last year	47
Santa Fe de Bogota, Columbia	1991–2	199 CSWs presenting for STD testing	78–95%	NS	All women participated in a study to evaluate the backup use of spermicides	48
Durban, South Africa	1991–2	12	25% never, 75% sometimes	0%		49
Bali, Indonesia	1992–3	614 variety of settings	19–90% (mean 35%)	0–11%	Lowest condom use (19%) in low priced workers	50
Bali, Indonesia	1992–3	80 males	48% anal receptive, 55% anal insertive, 17% oral receptive, 14% oral insertive	19% anal receptive, 33% anal insertive, 0% oral receptive and insertive		51
Surabaya, Indonesia	1992–3	187 variety of settings	14%–67%	NS	Condom use over the last week	52
La Paz, Bolivia	1992 1993 1994 1995	135 133 153 265	36.5% 38.8% 62.8% 72.5%	NS	Condoms use increased with behavioural intervention	53

Table 8.2 (continued)

Place	Date	Number, sex[a] and place of work	Percentage using condoms for commercial sex	Percentage using condoms with regular partners	Comments	Reference
Hong Kong	1993	190 STD clinic	38% always, 19% seldom or never	18% always, 55% seldom or never		54
Bali, Indonesia	1994	300 brothel	18–29% for vaginal sex in the day before, 62–75% after intervention. Control group 47% before and 60% after	1–13% for vaginal sex in the week before, 56–57% after intervention. Control group 20% before and 36% after	Intervention included education by outreach workers together with condom sales and distribution. No intervention in control group	55
Sungai Kolok, Betong, Thailand	1994	283 brothel	72–80% condom use	NS	No change with health promotion alone	56
4 cities in Thailand	1994–5	504 brothel	97–98% always for male or female condoms	NS	Women were divided into 2 groups: male condoms alone, or a combination of male and female condoms	57
Kramat Tunggak, Indonesaia	1995	459 brothel	25% never, 22% seldom, 17% often and 36% always	NS		58
Iloilo City, Indonesia	1995	110 registered and 42 freelance CSWs from bars and clubs	74% registered and 43% of freelance always and 15% registered and 38% freelance never	NS		59

[a] Female unless otherwise stated.
NS, not stated.

that there is no need for condoms at home.[62] Whilst the distinction between commercial and non-commercial sex may have some logic, some unpaid partners may have several other partners thus placing CSWs at risk for STIs and HIV.[2]

In contrast to the voluminous literature relating to condom use in the female sex industry, little is published about males and transsexuals who sell sex.[28,35,44,51,63] A study of 27 male commercial sex workers from Holland showed that 50 per cent used condoms for receptive anal sex and 25 per cent for insertive anal sex with male clients.[64] A large study from Thailand (1 172 males) found that condoms were used always by 58 per cent, whilst 42 per cent did not use condoms or used them inconsistently with male clients.[44] Studies of transvestites in Rome and Jakarta suggest that condoms are seldom used for commercial sex.[62,35]

Predictors of and barriers to condom use

Studies of CSWs and their clients have identified a number of predictors of consistent condom use. These include knowledge about AIDS and other STIs, level of self-esteem, perception of personal risk, perceptions about decrease or increase in pleasure with condom use, and the availability of condoms.[65,66]

In addition, many barriers to the use of condoms have been identified:

- financial difficulties
- education level of CSWs and/or clients
- homelessness
- social class of CSWs and/or clients
- violence, threats of violence or coercion towards the CSW by clients or pimps
- refusal by clients
- false perceptions about the need for condoms
- lack of availability
- sex with "regular" clients
- lack of community support
- lack of legal protection
- work conditions
- drug (including alcohol) use by the CSW and/or clients
- social context of commercial sex work
- working in a foreign or unfamiliar environment

- job satisfaction
- discomfort or pain associated with condom use and lack of lubrication
- appearance of client
- delay in ejaculation and unwanted prolongation of the sexual act.

Some of these (e.g. social class, financial difficulties, homelessness and lack of education) are related to socioeconomic factors within the community. Others, are a product of the complex interrelationship between CSWs, their clients, their non-paying partners and the community.

Vanwesenbeeck and co-workers studied risk-taking behaviour in 127 female CSWs in Holland. The women were classified on the basis of consistent condom use into three groups: "consistent protectors", "selective risk takers", and "risk takers". Using semi-structured interviews and a variety of questionnaires they identified a number of differences between the risk takers and others. The risk takers were more likely to have suffered victimisation as a child or adult, have low job satisfaction, the greatest financial need and the greatest stress.[67]

Considerable skill may be required in negotiating safer sex, particularly if there is client resistance or the threat of violence.[68] Many workers develop strategies using humour or the threat of STIs to encourage condom use[69] and some have developed sophisticated techniques to place a condom on the client's penis without their knowledge. Others refuse penetrative sex if the client declines to use a condom.[31]

CSWs working in brothels, stress the importance of a supportive management. However, those working alone particularly on the street, are sometimes threatened with violence or coercion.

In poorer communities financial considerations are often uppermost, with rural poverty driving many women towards commercial sex work. Lack of other employment opportunities are sometimes important in the decision not to use condoms[70] and the need for food, clothing or shelter often determines the personal decision or the decision by the brothel manager or pimp to use or not use condoms.[71,72]

In some parts of Africa, herbs and other agents are used to dry-up vaginal secretions. These agents are believed to enhance sexual pleasure and "dry sex" is used by some CSWs. This may result in a reluctance to use condoms in the belief that they may "block the magic" of the drying agents or that the use of condoms with dry sex may result in condom breakage.[73]

Female condoms

Female condoms offer an alternative method of protection for CSWs and their clients against STIs and HIV. Several studies have shown that in the context of commercial sex, female condoms offer an acceptable and largely problem-free alternative or adjunct to the male condom. A study among 51 female CSWs in Costa Rica reported that 51 per cent of the women "liked the female condom very much" and 45 per cent liked it somewhat. Over two-thirds preferred the female condom to the male equivalent and over half said that their clients preferred them.[74] Other studies have confirmed high satisfaction rates, although some workers felt that the appearance may deter clients.[75]

Promoting condom use

A number of the programmes promoting condom use within the sex industry (often linked with other health promotion and STD reduction strategies) have been highly successful. Most have increased condom use from very low levels to 80 per cent or above, and many have resulted in a dramatic decline in STIs in CSWs, their clients, and the general community.

One of the most successful programmes has been the so called "100 per cent condom program" in Thailand. In 1988 it became apparent that the commercial sex industry was playing a major role in fuelling the HIV epidemic. The government, through the extensive network of brothels, promoted the use of condoms by CSWs, brothel owners, and clients. In addition condoms were provided free of charge and there was an extensive media campaign.[60] As a result, condom use went from an estimated 14 per cent in 1982–9 to 93 per cent in 1993, and STI cases (syphilis, gonorrhoea, chancroid, lymphogranuloma venereum, and non-gonococcal urethritis) diagnosed in government STI clinics fell from over 237 000 in 1987 to just under 39 000 in 1993.[76]

Other successful campaigns have been conducted in numerous places including Nairobi Kenya, Kinshasa (formerly Zaire), Singapore, Honduras, Accra Ghana, Bali Indonesia, and India.[34,37,41,77–80] One common feature of these programmes is the provision and distribution of condoms.

Condom use can be sustained over several years, by close monitoring and prompt action to address problems or concerns, by continuing health promotion activities, by involving CSWs in all phases of the project and by the ongoing availability of condoms.[79]

Condom breakage and slippage

Condom breakage and slippage are uncommon in the commercial sex industry. In Holland CSWs self-reported a breakage rate of 0.8 per cent and clients a rate of 1.5 per cent. Some breaks were due to user error or action (e.g. exposure to oil-based lubricants, incorrect usage, sharp fingernails or teeth, rough sex, condom broken purposely by client) some to anatomical variations (e.g. large penis) and some due to the age or poor quality of the condom.[81] Slippage rates were also low: 0.1–0.9 per cent identified by CSWs and 0.2–1.3 per cent identified by clients. The identified reasons were similar to those identified for breakage. Very similar rates have been reported from Thailand (1.5 per cent breakage and 0.1 per cent slippage),[82] Nevada, USA (0 per cent breakage and 0.6 per cent slippage)[31] and Sydney, Australia (0.5 per cent breakage for vaginal sex and 0.8 per cent for anal sex).[83]

The availability of condoms of different sizes, use of new and good quality condoms, avoidance of oil-based lubricants, and increased awareness of the human factors responsible for some failures will further reduce the risk of breakage and slippage.

Conclusions

Condoms are widely used in the commercial sex industry, particularly in developed countries. Health promotion activities, including health information for CSWs and clients, and the availability of condoms have had a dramatic impact in increasing condom use and thereby improving personal and public health by decreasing the incidence of STIs. Failure rates in the industry are very low and could be reduced further by the availability of new, good quality condoms of various sizes. Low condom-use for non-paying partners is a potential source of STIs for CSWs and strategies for increasing condom use in this setting are required.

References

1 Coleman E. The development of male prostitution activity among gay and bisexual adolescents. *J Homosex* 1989; **17**: 131–49.

2 Day S and Ward H. Sex workers and the control of sexually transmitted disease. *Genitourin Med* 1997; **73**: 161–8.

3 Celentano DD, Nelson KE, Suprasert S, *et al.* Behavioural and sociodemographic risks for frequent visits to commercial sex workers among Northern Thai men. *AIDS* 1993; **12**: 1647–52.

4 Wellings K, Field J, Johnson A, Wadsworth J. *Sexual behaviour in Britain.* London: Penguin, 1994.

5 Piot P, Plummer FA, Rey MA, *et al.* Retrospective seroepidemiology of AIDS virus infection in Nairobi populations. *J Infect Dis* 1987; **155**: 1108–12.

6 Nzila N, Laga M, Thiam MA, *et al.* HIV and other sexually transmitted diseases among female prostitutes in Kinshasa. *AIDS* 1991; **5**: 715–21.

7 O'Connor CC, Berry G, Rohrsheim R, Donovan B. Sexual health and use of condoms among local and international sex workers in Sydney. *Genitourin Med* 1996; **72**: 47–51.

8 Yorke JA, Hethcote HW and Nold A. Dynamics and control of the spread of gonorrhoea. *Sex Trans Dis* 1978; **5**: 51–6.

9 Estcourt CS, Rorhrsheim R, Marks C, *et al.* Male commercial sex workers: HIV, STDs and risk behaviours. Abstract 103. Australian Society for HIV Medicine, 10th Annual Conference, Newcastle, Australia, 1998.

10 Elifson K, Boles J, Doll L. HIV seroprevalence and risk factors among clients of male and female prostitutes. VIII International conference on AIDS/III STD World Congress. Amsterdam, July 1992 (abstract POC 5616).

11 Morse E, Simon P, Osofsky H, Balson P, Gaumer H. The male street prostitute; a vector for the transmission of HIV infection into the heterosexual world. *Soc Sci Med* 1991; **32**: 535–9.

12 Weir SS, Roddy RE, Zeking L, Ryan KA, Wong El. Measuring condom use: asking "Do you or don't you" isn't enough. *AIDS Educ Prevent* 1998; **10**(4): 293–302.

13 Tchoudomirova K, Domeika M, Mårdh P-A. Demographic data on prostitutes from Bulgaria – a recruitment country for international (migratory) prostitutes. *Int J STD AIDS* 1997; **8**: 187–191.

14 Papaevangelou G, Roumeliotou A, Kallinikos, G, Papoutsakis G, Trichopoulou E, Stefanou Th. Eduaction in preventing HIV infection in Greek registered prostitutes. *J Acquir Immun Defic Syndr* 1988; 1(4): 386–9.

15 van den Hoek JAR, van Haastrecht HJA, Scheeringa-Troost B, Goudsmit J, Coutinho RA. HIV infection and STD in drug addicted prostitutes in Amsterdam: potential for heterosexual HIV transmission. *Genitourin Med* 1989; **65**: 146–50.

16 Seidlin M, Krasinski K, Bebenroth D, Itri V, Paolino AM, Valentine F. Prevalence of HIV infection in New York call girls. *J Acquir Immun Def Syndr Hum Retrovirol* 1988; **1**: 150–4.

17 Dorfman LE, Derish PA, Cohen JB. Hey Girlfriend: an evaluation of AIDS prevention among women in the sex industry. *Health Educ Q* 1992; **19**(1): 25–40.

18 Philpot CR, Harcourt CL, Edwards JM. A survey of female prostitutes at risk of HIV infection and other transmissible diseases. *Genitourin Med* 1991; **67**: 384–88.

19 van Ameijden EJ, van den Hoek AJ van Haastrescht HJ, Coutinho RA. Trends in sexual behaviour and the incidence of sexually transmitted diseases and HIV among drug-using prostitutes, Amsterdam 1986–1992. *AIDS* 1994; **8**: 213–21.

20 Mak RP, Plum JR. Do prostitutes need more health education regarding sexually transmitted diseases and the HIV infection? Experience in a Belgian city. *Soc Sci Med* 1991; **33**(8): 963–6.

21 Spina M, Mancuso S, Sinicco A, et al. Human immunodeficiency virus seroprevalence and condom use among female sex workers in Italy. *Sex Trans Dis* 1998; **25**(9): 451–4.

22 Ward H, Day S, Mezzone J, et al. Prostitution and risk of HIV: female prostitutes in London. *BMJ* 1993; **307**: 356–8.

23 Wong ML, Tan TC, Ho ML, Lim JY, Wan S, Chan R. Factors associated with sexually transmitted diseases among prostitutes in Singapore. *Int J STD AIDS* 1992; **3**: 332–7.

24 European Working Group on HIV Infection in Female Prostitutes. HIV infection in European female sex workers: epidemiological link with use of petroleum-based lubricants. *AIDS* 1993; **7**: 401–8.

25 Alary M, Worm A-M, Kvinesdal B. Risk behaviours for HIV infection and sexually transmitted diseases among female sex workers from Copenhagen. *Int J STD AIDS* 1994; **5**: 365–7.

26 Tanaka M, Nakayama H, Sakumoto M, Matsumoto T, Akazawa K, Kumazawa J. Trends in sexually transmitted diseases and condom use patterns among commercial sex workers in Fukuoka City, Japan 1990–3. *Genitourin Med* 1996; **72**: 358–61.

27 van Haastrecht HJ, Fennema JS, Coutinho RA, van der Helm TCM, Kint JAP, van den Hoek JAR. HIV prevalence and risk behaviour among prostitutes and clients in Amsterdam: migrants at increased risk for HIV infection. *Genitourin Med* 1993; **69**: 251–6.

28 Jones DL, Irwin KL, Inciardi J, et al. The high-risk sexual practices of crack-smoking sex workers recruited from the streets of three American cities. *Sex Trans Dis* 1998; **25**(4): 198–93.

29 Archibald CP, Chan RKW, Wong ML, Goh A, Goh CL. Evaluation of a safe-sex intervention programme among sex workers in Singapore. *Int J STD AIDS* 1994; **5**: 268–72.

30 Pyett PM, Haste BR, Snow JD. Who works in the sex industry? A profile of female prostitutes in Victoria. *Austral N Z J Public Health* 1996; **20**(4): 431–3.

31 Albert AE, Warner DL, Hatcher RA, Trussell J, Bennett C. Condom use among female commercial sex workers in Nevada's legal brothels. *Am J Public Health* 1995; **85**(11): 1514–20.

32 Strang J, Powis B, Griffiths P, Gossop M. Heterosexual vaginal and anal intercourse amongst London heroin and cocaine users. *In J STD AIDS* 1994; **5**: 133–6.

33 Swaddiwudhipong W, Chaovakiratipong C, Siri S, Lerdlukanavonge P. Sociodemographic characteristics and incidence of gonorrhoea in prostitutes working near the Thai–Burmese border. *Southeast Asian J Trop Med Public Health* 1990; **21**(1): 45–52.

34 Laga M, Alary M, Nzila N, et al. Condom promotion, sexually transmitted diseases treatment, and declining incidence of HIV-1 infection in female Zairian sex workers. *Lancet* 1994; **344**: 246–8.

35 Lubis I, Master J, Bambang M, Papilaya A, Anthony RL. AIDS related attitudes and sexual practices of the Jakarta Waria (male transvestites). *Southeast Asian J Trop Med Public Health* 1994; **25**(1): 102–6.

36 Mann JM, Nzilambi N, Piot P, et al. HIV infection and associated risk factors in female prostitutes in Kinshasa, Zaire. *AIDS* 1988; **2**: 249–54.

37 Ngugi EN, Plummer FA, Simonsen JN, et al. Prevention of transmission of human immunodeficiency virus in Africa: effectiveness of condom promotion and health education among prostitutes. *Lancet* 1988; **2** (8616): 887–90.

38 Kanki P, M'Boup S, Marlink R, et al. Prevalence and risk determinants of human immunodeficiency virus type 2 (HIV-2) and human immunodeficiency

virus type 1 (HIV-1) in West African female prostitutes. *Am J Epidemiol* 1992; **136**(7): 895–907.

39 Golenbock DT, Guerra J, Pfister J, *et al.* Absence of infection with human immunodeficiency virus in Peruvian prostitutes. *AIDS Res Hum Retrovir* 1988; 4(6): 493–9.

40 Cameron DW, Ngugi EN, Ronald AR, *et al.* Condom use prevents genital ulcers in women working as prostitutes. *Sex Trans Dis* 1991; **18**(3): 188–91.

41 Asamoah-Adu A, Weir S, Pappoe M, Kanlisi N, Neequaye A, Lamptey P. Evaluation of a targeted AIDS prevention intervention to increase condom use among prostitutes in Ghana. *AIDS* 1994; 8(2): 239–46.

42 Pickering H, Quigley M, Hayes RJ, Todd J, Wilkins A. Determinants of condom use in 24,000 prostitute/client contacts in The Gambia. *AIDS* 1993; 7(8): 1093–8.

43 Ngugi EN, Wilson D, Scbstad J, Plummer FA, Moses S. Focused peer-mediated educational programs among female sex workers to reduce sexually transmitted disease and human immunodeficiency virus transmission in Kenya and Zimbabwe. *J Infect Dis* 1996; 174(Suppl 2): S240–7.

44 Kunawararak P, Beyrer C, Natpratan C, *et al.* The epidemiology of HIV and syphilis among male commercial sex workers in nothern Thailand. *AIDS* 1995; **5**: 517–21.

45 Sakondhavat C, Werawatanakul Y, Bennett A, Kuchaisit C, Suntharapa S. Promoting condom-only brothels through solidarity and support for brothel managers. *Int J STD AIDS* 1997; **8**: 40–3.

46 Lurie P, Fernandes MEL, Hughes V, *et al.* Socioeconomic status and risk of HIV-1, syphilis and hepatitis B infection among sex workers in São Paulo State, Brazil. *AIDS* 1995; 9(Suppl 1): S31–7.

47 Sánchez J, Gotuzzo E, Escamilla J, *et al.* Sexually transmitted infections in female sex workers: reduced by condom use but not by a limited periodic examination program. *Sex Trans Dis* 1998; 25(2): 82–9.

48 Farr G, Castro LAA, DiSantostcfano MS, Claassen E, Olguin F. Use of spermicide and impact of prophylactic condom use among sex workers in Santa Fe de Botota, Colombia. *Sex Trans Dis* 1996; 23(3): 206–11.

49 Karim QA, Karim SSA, Soldan K, Zondi M. Reducing the risk of HIV infection among South African sex workers: socioeconomic and gender barriers. *Am J Public Health* 1995; 85(11): 1521–5.

50 Ford K, Wirawan DN, Fajans P. AIDS knowledge, risk behaviours, and condom use among four groups of female sex workers in Bali, Indonesia. *J Acquir Immun Defic Syndr Hum Retrovirol* 1995; 10(5): 569–76.

51 Ford K, Wirawan DN, Fajans P, Thorpe L. AIDS knowledge, risk behaviours, and factors related to condom use among male commercial sex workers and male tourist clients in Bali, Indonesia. *AIDS* 1995; 9: 751–9.

52 Joesoef MR, Linnan M, Barakbah Y, Idajadi A, Kambodji A, Schulz K. Patterns of sexually transmitted diseases in female sex workers in Surabaya, Indonesia. *Int J STD AIDS* 1997; **8**: 576–80.

53 Levine WC, Revollo R, Kaune V, *et al.* Decline in sexually transmitted disease prevalence in female Bolivian sex works: impact of an HIV prevention project. *AIDS* 1998; **12**: 1899–906.

54 Wong KH, Lee SS, Lo YC, Lo KK. Condom use among female commercial sex workers and male clients in Hong Kong. *Int J STD AIDS* 1994; 5: 287–9.

55 Ford K, Wirawan DN, Fajans P, Meliawan P, MacDonald K, Thorpe L. Behavioral interventions for reduction of sexually transmitted disease/HIV transmission among female commercial sex workers and clients in Bali, Indonesia. *AIDS* 1996; **10**: 213–22.

56 van Griensven GJP, Limanonda B, Ngaokeow S, Ayuthaya SIN, Poshyachinda V. Evaluation of a targeted HIV prevention programme among female commercial sex workers in the south of Thailand. *Sex Transm Inf* 1998; 74: 54–8.

57 Fontanet AL, Saba J, Chandelying V, et al. Protection against sexually transmitted diseases by granting sex workers in Thailand the choice of using the male or female condom: results from a randomized controlled trial. AIDS 1998; 12(14): 1851–9.

58 Sedyaningsih-Mamahit ER, Gortmaker SL. Determinants of safer-sex behaviors of brothel female commercial sex workers in Jakarta, Indonesia. J Sex Res 1999; 36(2): 190–7.

59 Liu TI, So R. Knowledge, attitude, and prevention practice survey regarding AIDS comparing registered to freelance commercial sex workers in Iloilo City, Philippines. Southeast Asian J Trop Med Public Health 1996; 27(4): 696–702.

60 Rojanapithayakorn W, Hanenberg R. The 100% condom program in Thailand. AIDS 1996; 10: 1–7.

61 Cusick L. Non-use of condoms by prostitute women. AIDS Care 1998; 10(2): 133–46.

62 Pyett PM, Warr DJ. Vulnerability on the streets: female sex workers and HIV risk. AIDS Care 1997; 9(5): 539–47.

63 Gattari P, Spizzichino C, Valenzi M, Saccarelli M, Rezza G. Behavioural patterns and HIV infection among drug using transvestites practising prostitution in Rome. AIDS Care 1992; 4(1) L83–7.

64 de Graaf R, Vanwesenbeeck I, van Zessen G, Straver CJ, Visser JH. Male prostitutes and safe sex: different settings, different risks. AIDS Care 1994; 6(3): 277–88.

65 Sohn M, Jin K. AIDS-related perceptions and condom use of prostitutes in Korea. Yonsei Med J 1999; 40(1): 9–13.

66 Thorpe L, Ford K, Fajans P, Wirawan DN. Correlates of condom use among female prostitutes and tourist clients in Bali, Indonesia. AIDS Care 1997; 9(2): 181–97.

67 Vanwesenbeeck I, de Graaf R, van Zessen G, Straver CJ, Visser JH. Professional HIV risk taking, levels of victimization, and well-being in female prostitutes in The Netherlands. Arch Sex Behav 1995; 24(5): 503–15.

68 Varga CA. The condom conundrum: barriers to condom use among commercial sex workers in Durban, South Africa. African J Reprod Health 1997; 1(1): 74–88.

69 Vanwesenbeeck I, van Zessen G, de Graaf R, Straver CJ. Contextual and interactional factors influencing condom use in heterosexual prostitution contacts. Pat Educ Counsel 1994; 24(3): 307–22.

70 Estabanez P, Rua-Figueroa M, Aguilar MD, Bru F, Zunzunegui M, Rog Emilio V. Condom use in clients of prostitutes in Spain. AIDS 1996; 10(4): 445–6.

71 Wawer MJ, Podhisita C, Kanungsukkasem U, Pramualratana A, McNamara R. Origins and working conditions of female sex workers in urban Thailand: consequences or social context for HIV transmission. Soc Sci Med 1996; 42(3): 453–62.

72 Bhave G, Lindan CP, Hudes ES, et al. Impact of an intervention on HIV, sexually transmitted diseases, and condom use among sex workers in Bombay, India. AIDS 1995; 8(Suppl 1): S21–30.

73 Civic D, Wilson D. Dry sex in Zimbabwe and implications for condom use. Soc Sci Med 1995; 42(1): 91–8.

74 Madrigal J, Schiffer J, Feldblum PJ. Female condom acceptability among sex workers in Costa Rica. AIDS Educ Prevent 1998; 10(20): 105–12.

75 Pyarat S, Verapool C, Steven S, Charn U. Perceptions and acceptability of the female condom (Femidom®) amongst commercial sex workers in the Songkla province, Thailand. Int J STD AIDS 1998; 9(3): 168–72.

76 Hanenberg RS, Rojanapithayakorn W, Kunasol P, Sokal DC. Impact of Thailand's HIV-control programme as indicated by the decline of sexually transmitted diseases. Lancet 1994; 344: 243–5.

77 Ford K, Wirawan DN, Fajans P, Thorpe L. AIDS knowledge, risk behaviours and factors related to condom use among male commercial sex workers and male tourist clients in Bali, Indonesia. *AIDS* 1995; **8**: 751–9.

78 Fox LJ, Bailey PE, Clarke-Martínez KL, Coello M, Ordoñez FN, Barahona F. Condom use among high-risk women in Honduras: evaluation of an AIDS prevention program. *AIDS Educ Prevent* 1993; **5**(1): 1–10.

79 Wong ML, Chan KWR, Koh D. A sustainable behavioral intervention to increase condom use and reduce gonorrohea among sex workers in Singapore: 2-year follow-up. *Prevent Med* 1998; **27**: 891–900.

80 Bentley ME, Spratt K, Shepherd ME, *et al*. HIV testing and counseling among men attending sexually transmitted disease clinics in Pune, India: changes in condom use and sexual behavior over time. *AIDS* 1998; **12**: 1869–77.

81 de Graaf R, Vanwesenbeeck I, van Zessen G, Straver CJ, Visser JH. The effectiveness of condom use in heterosexual prostitution in The Netherlands. *AIDS* 1993; **7**: 265–9.

82 Rugpao S, Beyrer C, Tovanabutra S, *et al*. Multiple condom use and decreased condom breakage and slippage in Thailand. *J Acquir Immun Def Syndr Hum Retrovirol* 1997; **14**: 169–73.

83 Richters J, Donovan B, Gerofi J, Watson L. Low condom breakage rate in commercial sex. *Lancet* 1998; **24**: 31.

9 Condoms for anal sex

JULIET RICHTERS, SUSAN KIPPAX

Anal intercourse is associated in many people's minds with male homosexuality. However, some male homosexuals do not have anal intercourse, and some heterosexuals do.

Discussion of anal intercourse in the sexological literature has been very limited.[1] Even Kinsey, who was usually extremely broad-minded and non-judgmental about sexual practices, including bestiality and paedophilia, paid it very little attention. In *Sexual Behavior in the Human Male*[2] he concedes the lack of any need for a special theory to explain anal eroticism – it is from a physiological point of view unremarkable that people might enjoy it. Yet his discussion of anal sex is curiously truncated, only two paragraphs in the 800-page book. The scientific silence around anal sex continued until the advent of AIDS, which resulted in a burst of research and writing around the risks of anal sex for HIV transmission and the promotion of condom use by homosexually active men. This has not been matched by sexological attention to anal sex as a practice, with the exception of a few papers designed to inform health professionals (who are presumed to be personally unacquainted with anal eroticism) about such practices.[3,4] In striking contrast, a more recent paper regards pain during anal intercourse as a sexual dysfunction.[5]

Issues specific to the use of condoms for anal sex have remained little studied. This neglect is reflected in the lack of evidence for some of the major questions that are considered in this chapter, for example whether a stronger condom is required for anal than for vaginal intercourse.

132

How many people have anal intercourse?

The term "anal sex" is used in this chapter to mean penetrative penile–anal intercourse, not including rimming (oral–anal sex) or other anal erotic behaviour.

Heterosexuals

The British National Survey of Sexual Attitudes and Lifestyles reported that among men aged 16–59, 14 per cent had ever tried heterosexual anal sex, 6.5 per cent had practised it in the last year and 1.7 per cent in the last week. Among women, the figures were slightly lower (consistent with lower reporting of most sexual acts and number of partners by women): 13 per cent said they had ever had anal sex, 5.9 per cent in the last year, and 1.2 per cent in the last week.[6]

The United States national survey done at the same time had a considerably smaller sample size, so some of its subcategory estimates are less reliable, but it appears that anal sex is somewhat more prevalent in America. Among men aged 18–59, 25.6 per cent reported ever having had anal sex. Of those who had ever had a sexual experience, 9.6 per cent had practised anal sex in the last year and 2.3 per cent had practised anal sex as part of their last sexual event. Among women, 20.4 per cent reported having ever had anal sex, 8.6 per cent had done so in the past year and 1.2 per cent at their last sexual event.[7] These figures are consistent with the findings of Voeller's exhaustive review of 200+ studies reporting heterosexual anal intercourse and/or female anal STIs[1] Although bisexual men are more likely than exclusively heterosexual men to practise anal sex with women, the majority of heterosexual anal sex cannot be attributed to them. A telephone survey of Californians found that among heterosexuals (excluding those who had had any same-sex contact), 8 per cent of men and 6 per cent of women reported having anal sex at least once a month in the past year.[8]

There are many other national surveys of sexual behaviour, but most do not report anal intercourse separately; some do not even ask the question. For example, the ACSF Investigators in France report that they did not define the term "sexual intercourse" in their questionnaire.[9]

Anal intercourse is thus a minority practice among heterosexuals. Furthermore, people who have tried it do not necessarily take it up into their regular sexual repertoire. They may try it and find they dislike it, or they may reserve it for special occasions or particular partners. Anal sex differs in this respect from oral sex: people who have tried oral sex at all usually adopt it as part of their usual sexual repertoire.[7] It is less likely to be practised with casual partners[7] and generally attracts a premium when it is offered by female sex workers.[10]

Homosexual men

In the US survey, 27 per cent of men who reported any same-sex sexual behaviour, desire *or* identity (i.e. identified as gay, bisexual etc. – there were 150 such men, representing 10.1 per cent of the sample) had engaged in insertive anal sex with other men since puberty, and 29 per cent reported receptive anal sex. Among men who had had any male partners in the past year (2.7 per cent of the total sample), 79 per cent had had insertive anal sex and 77 per cent receptive.[7] Thus anal intercourse is very common but not universal among American men who are currently homosexually active.

In the UK survey, among men who reported any genital contact with men (3.6 per cent of the total sample), 34 per cent had ever had insertive anal intercourse with a man and 35 per cent had had receptive anal sex.[6] As "any genital contact" is a more limiting definition of homosexual activity than "any same-sex behaviour, desire or identity", we would expect a higher proportion of these men to have had anal sex if this practice were as prevalent in the UK as in the USA. Unfortunately, the UK survey does not report experience of anal sex in the last year as a percentage of those reporting any male partners in the past year for direct comparison.

In Australia, no national sample survey of sexual practices has yet been carried out although one is currently in development. A national non-random phone-in survey about male-to-male sex found that in 1996 around 80 per cent of respondents (men who had had at least one male partner in the past five years) had had anal sex in the past six months.[11] In a Sydney convenience-sample survey of men recruited at gay venues and events (also men who had had at least one male partner in the past five years), 84 per cent had had any anal intercourse in the past six months.[12] Such non-random surveys tend to include fewer homosexually active men who do not regard themselves as gay, or who have no contact with a gay community.

These survey results, together with clinical data and data from qualitative and small-scale studies of sexual practice, indicate that anal intercourse is not a universal male homosexual practice, but a very common one, particularly in established gay communities such as those of Europe,[13] the English-speaking countries and the Americas. It is commoner among men in gay relationships and less common in casual sex.[14] Among homosexually active men who are not attached to gay communities and may identify as heterosexual, anal intercourse (and indeed other anal erotic practices) appears to be somewhat less common as a sexual practice.[11] This is also true of homosexually active men in countries such as China where there are not large urban gay communities.[15,16]

Condoms and anal sex

Heterosexual couples in established relationships rarely use condoms for disease prevention unless one partner is known to be infected with herpes or HIV[17] (or, presumably, has some other STI, though evidence on this is sparse). Heterosexual couples have more often used condoms for pregnancy prevention, which is not an issue with anal intercourse; indeed anal intercourse may be used (like *coitus interruptus*) as a fertility-control practice,[18] or as a technique for the preservation of technical virginity.[1] The use of condoms for anal sex by heterosexual couples, or by the clients of female sex workers, has been little discussed. Most health promotion material aimed at heterosexuals either ignores anal sex altogether, because of a desire to avoid offence,[19] or brackets it without comment with vaginal sex, as in "Always use condoms for vaginal or anal sex".

Although more acts of anal intercourse are performed by heterosexual couples than between men,[1] research into the use of condoms for anal intercourse has been almost entirely occupied with homosexually active men. This emphasis is doubtless due to discomfort with heterosexual anal intercourse as a topic, but is also partially justified because anal intercourse between men is riskier owing to the higher prevalence of HIV infection in gay communities.

Condom use by homosexual men

Despite their honourable history for disease prevention, particularly in commercial sex, condoms did not become part of usual sexual practice in the developing homosexual communities of the 1970s. Not until gay communities responded to AIDS in the mid-1980s did they become an expected part of homosexual sex.

The early proposals in the mid-1980s to recommend condom use were pragmatic: there was no clear high-quality evidence that condoms would be effective against whatever caused AIDS, but the idea that AIDS would turn out to be caused by a transmissible pathogen and thus preventable by mechanical means seemed plausible – and promoting condom use seemed better than doing nothing. At the very least it would help reduce the high incidence of curable STIs in gay communities. Gay men in the United States, the United Kingdom, Australia and New Zealand and many countries in western Europe began to use condoms in order to protect themselves. While some gay communities were quick to take up condoms – gay men in New York, for example, coining the term "safe/safer sex" in 1982, before HIV had been discovered – others took more time, for example gay men in the Netherlands.

Objections were raised at the time, however.[20] Some of them were clearly the product of a general pre-existing prejudice against harm-minimisation in sexual medicine by people who preferred moral exhortation along the lines of "just say no" as an STI preventive.[21,22] Another, which has survived in various forms since then, is the idea that anal intercourse is rougher than vaginal sex and therefore that ordinary condoms would not withstand the special stresses of anal intercourse. This is an empirical question which is discussed below.

Prevalence of condom usage

How many homosexually active men use condoms when they have anal sex? Measurements of use vary between studies, but all show that in most western gay communities men have accepted condom use as a necessary part of HIV risk management.[13,14] In a large Canadian survey, of 2780 men who reported anal intercourse in the three months preceding the survey, 86 per cent used condoms at least on some occasions and 14 per cent never used them.[23] In Australia, of 2422 men who reported anal intercourse in the preceding six months, 82 per cent used a condom at least on some occasions.[11] In New Zealand, of 811 men who reported anal sex with a casual partner, 86 per cent used a condom at least sometimes, and 54 per cent of those reporting anal sex with a regular partner used condoms at least sometimes.[24] (All these studies used similar questionnaires by telephone, so they are comparable. All used convenience sampling, so the usual caveats must be made about generalising beyond the kind of men likely to respond to recruitment through gay communities.)

The difference between behaviour with regular and casual partners observed in New Zealand is seen in other surveys where the information has been sought. Like heterosexuals, homosexual men commonly abandon condom use in ongoing relationships when they perceive the risk of infection from the regular partner to be low. When accompanied by ascertainment of HIV seronegativity in both partners and an explicit arrangement about sex outside the relationship (for example no sex, no anal sex, or sex only with condoms), this strategy is called negotiated safety.[14]

How effective are condoms at preventing STI transmission during anal sex?

Evidence on the effectiveness *in vitro* of condoms in preventing transmission of sexually transmissible pathogens including HIV is given in Chapter 5.

Infection despite diligent use may arise from contamination by semen or other bodily fluids before or after intercourse, by late application of the condom,[25] by removal during intercourse,[26] or by mechanical failure of the condom, i.e. leakage, tearing (usually called breakage) or slipping off. Leakage through holes is thought to be rare with modern condoms (see Chapter 2).

When condom use was first proposed by gay communities responding to AIDS, many gay men were unfamiliar with condoms, or remembered them from perhaps unsatisfactory heterosexual episodes in the past. The high breakage rates and other difficulties recorded in early studies of condom use by gay men reflected this unfamiliarity.[27-29]

Breakage and slippage rates for condoms used in anal sex are shown in Tables 9.1 and 9.2. Bear in mind that study designs vary greatly, as do ways of measuring failure events and condom use. Some studies exclude breakage on application, or events judged to be due to certain categories of "incorrect use". Slippage is generally defined as the condom completely slipping off the penis. Experienced users may deal with partial slippage by adjusting the condom manually during sex, so slippage results may not always

Table 9.1 Condom breakage rate studies, anal sex

Study	Year	Study design	Breakage rate (%)	Number broken/ number used	User population
van Griensven et al., 1988[32]	1986	Retro	2.7	40/1468	112 homosexual men, Netherlands
Wigersma and Oud, 1987[28]	≤ 1987	Pro	10.5	21/200	17 homosexual couples, Netherlands, no regular condom users
Tindall et al., 1989[33]	1987	Retro	4.6–7.3 / 5.1–5.4	Not stated	Homosexually active men, Sydney (158 men reporting insertive use, 147 receptive)
Thompson et al., 1993[34]	1987	Retro	< 3[a]	Not stated	741 gay men, New York
Richters et al., 1988[35]	1988	Pro	0.5	3/664	30 male prostitutes, Sydney
Golombok et al., 1989[36]	1988	Retro	4.7[b]	Not stated	97 homosexually active men, London
Weinstock et al., 1993[39]	1989	Retro	4.2	1/24	Heterosexual STD clinic clients, San Francisco
Richters et al., 1993[37]	1989	Retro	8.0	523/6574	172 homosexually active clinic clients, Sydney
Sparrow and Lavill, 1994[38]	1992	Pro	32	6/19	540 family planning clinic clients[c]
Golombok et al., 1994[40]	≤ 1994	Pro	1.8	14/772	86 gay men, London
Benton et al., 1997[41]	1996	Pro	2.7	13/482	92 male volunteers, mostly experienced condom users[d]

[a] Breakage and slippage combined into failure rate of 3.3% (insertive) and 2.7% (receptive). [b] 5.3% for those using 5 to 50 condoms. [c] Of whom only a few (≤19) had anal intercourse. [d] No distinction is made between heterosexual and homosexual anal sex; there were 92 men in the study as a whole, with 1917 instances of condom use. Pro, prospective; Retro, retrospective.

Table 9.2 Condom slippage rate studies, anal sex

Study	Year	Study design	Slippage rate (%)	Number slipped of/number used	User population
van Griensven et al., 1988[32]	1986	Retro	5.2	71/1468	112 homosexual men, Netherlands
Wigersma and Oud, 1987[28]	≤ 1987	Pro	15.0	30/200	17 homosexual couples, Netherlands, no regular condom users
Thompson et al., 1993[34]	1987	Retro	< 3%[a]	Not stated	741 gay men, New York
Golombok et al., 1989[36]	1988	Retro	3.8[b]	Not stated	97 homosexually active men, London
Richters et al., 1993[37]	1989	Retro	5.1	336/6574	172 homosexually active clinic clients, Sydney
Sparrow and Lavill, 1994[38]	1992	Pro	32	6/19	540 family planning clinic clients[c]
Golombok et al., 1994[40]	≤ 1994	Pro	6.6[d]	51/772[d]	86 gay men, London

[a] Breakage and slippage combined into failure rate of 3.3% (insertive) and 2.7% (receptive). [b] 5.3% for those using 5 to 50 condoms. [c] Of whom only a few (≤19) had anal intercourse. [d] Slippage occurred during withdrawal on 28 of the 51 occasions. Pro, prospective; Retro, retrospective.

reflect the tendency of the condom to slip. Prospective experimental studies, where the condoms are distributed to the respondents and their exact number is known, are likely to produce more accurate figures, but the conditions of use may be more artificial. Proposals for more readily comparable study designs should be heeded by future researchers.[30,31]

Reasons for failure

The clearest finding is that experience with condoms reduces failure rates.[26,34,36,38,41,42] This would explain the very low breakage rates among sex workers[35] and the high rates found in both Wigersma and Oud's early study on 17 gay couples,[28] none of whom were regular condom users, and possibly Sparrow and Lavill's study.[38] The design of this study and the high breakage rate encourage the speculation that participants tried anal intercourse with a condom for the first time especially for the study. Very small numbers in the two studies of heterosexuals[38,39] mean that rate estimates are very unreliable.

Although research around the world has demonstrated the association of unprotected anal intercourse with transmission of HIV and other sexually transmitted pathogens, there are no cohort studies of sero-discordant male couples from which the degree of protection afforded by condom use can be estimated. Studies of heterosexual HIV-sero-discordant couples, in which anal and vaginal sex are not always clearly delineated, show about 85 per cent protection.[17,43,44] (See Chapter 5.)

Use of additional lubricant

Anal sex requires additional lubricant.[45] Oil-based lubricants damage condoms.[46] In 1989, Voeller suggested that inappropriate lubricant use was a major reason for high condom breakage rates among gay men, often because men mistook hand lotions, baby oil and other cremes for water-based because they wash off in water.[47] At the same time in Sydney, we found that few gay men used oil-based lubricants; it seems the message from the AIDS councils had been heard by men in the gay community.[26] Heterosexuals need to know that using extra lubricant reduces slippage in anal sex, although it may increase the risk for vaginal sex.[45]

Other issues

Many other issues – such as user characteristics (including penis size) and condom thickness, size and shape – apply to vaginal use just as much as anal use and are covered in Chapters 2, 3 and 11. Manufacturers have been slow to make condoms available in a range of sizes, even though a proportion of respondents to research into condom attitudes have always complained that they found condoms too wide, tight or short.[27,48,49] (See Chapter 2.)

Are special stronger condoms required for anal sex?

This was a question much asked in the mid-1980s in the early days of AIDS and safe sex. It is claimed that anal intercourse involves greater friction.[28] As the lining of the rectum is considerably less tough than the lining of the vagina, it could be argued that this claim is nothing more than a transfer of masculine symbolism onto the material world. Men may break condoms with their rough horny fingers, or their rough thrusting, more than women with their soft little hands, or their gentle romantic intercourse. Yet women's long nails and rings have also been under suspicion in the past. Cock rings and penile piercings, fashionable in some gay communities, could also pose a risk to condoms. Such arguments are no more than supposition.

In their 1997 review, Silverman and Gross argue that "there is uncertainty as to the level of protection that condoms designed for use during VI (vaginal intercourse) can provide during AI (anal intercourse)".[50] This overestimates the specificity of condom design. Historically, condoms may have been used largely for vaginal intercourse, but they cannot be said to have been "designed" for it. The condom is a latex reproduction or imitation of a butcher's by-product, the traditional sheath made of the blind-ended, roughly cylindrical lamb caecum (a pouch at the beginning of the large intestine), which comes in a range of sizes which happen to fit the human penis. Variations in condom manufacture such as shaping, colour, teat ends, spots and stripes etc. are largely arbitrary marketing gimmicks. Testing of condoms is based on theoretical integrity of the condom: freedom from holes, tensile strength of the latex, etc. Tests were developed before any attempt was made to correlate their results with successful use *in vivo*.[51–54] (See Chapter 3.) Only empirical testing comparing similar populations of men using condoms for anal or vaginal sex (or, ideally, both) will tell us whether anal sex is tougher on condoms than vaginal sex.

Wigersma and Oud's study with 17 gay couples tested different condom types experimentally and found slightly higher failure rates in anal sex for ordinary condoms than for thicker stiffer ones. However, users disliked the stiffer (i.e. less distensible) ones the most.[28] Van Griensven et al. found a lower failure rate among those men surveyed who chose to use special anal condoms, but (as they admit) this is confounded by the possibility that the more careful men who chose the recommended "anal" condom would have had lower failure rates even if the condoms were in fact identical.[32] Some years later Golombok and Sheldon tested the failure rate of thicker condoms but without a comparison group using ordinary ones.[40] They argued (or perhaps their ethics committee argued) that it was "considered unethical" to provide gay men with condoms "which may have a high(er?) breakage rate". Evidence for their conclusion that a "thicker condom offers greater protection" is weak, especially as the time difference between their work and the earlier studies in 1988–9 means that more men in their sample would have been experienced condom users.

A recent cross-over trial of two types of condom showed that the stronger one was less likely to break in anal sex but slightly (non-significantly) more likely to break in oral and vaginal sex.[41] As multiple comparisons were made, and the sample using condoms for anal sex was smaller, the authors conclude that replication of their result is necessary.

It does appear in general that condom failure rates are somewhat higher for anal sex than for vaginal sex in similar groups of men. However, the difference is not nearly as large as that between different groups. In general, inexperienced users, less educated users and, in the USA, African-American men have higher failure rates. These are also the very groups with lower rates of condom use. Heavily recommending the use of special condoms for anal sex may lead men to feel that ordinary condoms are useless. Labelling condom packets "Intended for vaginal use only" may have the same effect.

At present, men who identify as heterosexual and require condoms for anal sex with either male or female partners can simply buy ordinary condoms. To provide separate and identifiable "anal" condoms would make condom purchase more difficult and stigmatising than it already is for such men. For men outside gay communities this is impractical. Furthermore, the user acceptability of a stiffer, thicker condom must be weighed against its theoretical effectiveness. The most ineffective condom is the one that is not used.

Issues around condom use for gay men and other men who have sex with men

Physical issues

Many condom users complain that they cannot get or maintain an erection while applying or wearing a condom, or that their ejaculation is delayed or premature (through constriction by the condom).[36,26] Such effects on sexual pleasure and function are considerable disincentives for condom use, especially in casual sex where performance pressure may be great.

Contextual issues

Many of the issues surrounding condom use for gay or homosexually active men have to do with the social context of the sexual activity rather than with the physiology of anal sex. Practical issues around condom provision arise in locations such as gay saunas and sex-on-premises venues where men may take part in anal sex with casual partners in dimly lit surroundings.[55] In the ideal venue, free condoms and lube are available in each cubicle, not just given singly to each man as he enters the venue. This is particularly important in saunas, where patrons enter the sauna wearing only a towel and cannot easily carry condoms with them. In some jurisdictions, such venues are illegal and managers are loath to provide condoms or even have them on the premises in case they are seized as evidence in police raids. Changing the law is then an important public health goal. The same difficulty may arise with condom use at public sex locations such as lavatories and parks (beats, cottages or tearooms) in countries where consenting male-to-male sex is illegal. Because of the danger of police harassment, men seeking sexual partners may avoid carrying condoms.

The adoption of other strategies to avoid HIV infection such as partner selection, negotiated safety, avoidance of anal intercourse, and avoidance of ejaculation all indicate dislike of condoms. Few men find them erotic or pleasurable, and most would rather not use them. Nonetheless, condoms continue to be used as a means of preventing HIV and STD transmission. The decline of HIV in countries where they have been promoted speaks to their efficacy.

References

1 Voeller B. AIDS and heterosexual anal intercourse. *Arch Sex Behav* 1991; **20**: 233–76.
2 Kinsey AC, Pomeroy WB, Martin CE. *Sexual behavior in the human male.* Philadelphia: WB Saunders, 1948: 579.
3 Agnew J. Some anatomical and physiological aspects of anal sexual practices. *J Homosex* 1985; **12**: 75–96.
4 Agnew J. Hazards associated with anal erotic activity. *Arch Sex Behav* 1986; **15**: 307–14.
5 Rosser BRS, Short BJ, Thurmes PJ, Coleman E. Anodyspareunia, the unacknowledged sexual dysfunction: a validation study of painful receptive anal intercourse and its psychosexual concomitants in homosexual men. *J Sex Marital Ther* 1998; **24**: 281–92.
6 Johnson A, Wadsworth J, Wellings K, Field J. *Sexual attitudes and lifestyles.* Oxford: Blackwell Scientific, 1994.
7 Laumann EO, Gagnon JH, Michael RT, Michaels S. *The social organization of sexuality: sexual practices in the United States.* Chicago and London: University of Chicago Press, 1994.
8 Erickson PI, Bastani R, Maxwell AE, Marcus AC, Capell FJ, Yan KX. Prevalence of anal sex among heterosexuals in California and its relationship to other AIDS risk factors. *AIDS Educ Prev* 1995; 7: 477–93.
9 ACSF Investigators (Spira A, Bajos N, Béjin A *et al.*). AIDS and sexual behaviour in France. *Nature* 1992; **360**: 407–9.
10 Perkins R, Bennett G. *Being a prostitute: prostitute women and prostitute men.* Sydney: George Allen Unwin, 1985: 225–7.
11 Crawford J, Kippax S, Rodden P, Donohoe S, Van de Ven P. *Male Call 96: national telephone survey of men who have sex with men.* Sydney: National Centre in HIV Social Research, 1998.
12 Knox S, Van de Ven P, Richters J, Prestage G, Crawford J, Kippax S. *Sydney gay community surveillance report no. 7: update to June 1998.* Sydney: National Centre in HIV Social Research, 1998.
13 Bochow M, Schiltz MA. Reactions of gay men to condom use in France and Germany. *XI International Conference on AIDS, Vancouver, July 7–12, 1996. Volume 2: Abstracts.* Abstract We.C.3483.
14 Kippax S, Connell RW, Dowsett GW, Crawford J. *Sustaining safe sex: gay communities respond to AIDS.* London: Falmer Press, 1993.
15 Pan S, Wu J, Gil VE. Homosexual behaviors in contemporary China. *J Psychol Hum Sex* 1995; 7(4): 1–17.
16 Williams WL. Asking the right questions: use of qualitative research to understand the social context and meanings of sexual behaviors cross-culturally, to develop safer-sex messages within diverse cultural groups. Paper presented to HIV Prevention Research Development Meeting sponsored by the CDC in conjunction with the National Lesbian/Gay Health Conference, Minneapolis, 18–19 June 1995. Department of Anthropology, University of Southern California.
17 De Vincenzi I, for the European Study Group on Heterosexual Transmission of HIV. A longitudinal study of human immunodeficiency virus transmission by heterosexual partners. *N Engl J Med* 1994; **331**: 341–6.

18 van de Walle E, Muhsam HV. Fatal secrets and the French fertility transition. *Pop Devel Rev* 1995; **21**: 261–79.
19 Wilton T. Safety in Pornutopia: desire, pleasure and safer sex education. Paper presented at HIV, AIDS and Society conference, "Social Science: From Theory to Practice", Macquarie University, Sydney, July 1995.
20 Gøtzsche PC, Hørding M. Condoms to prevent HIV transmission do not imply truly safe sex. *Scand J Infect Dis* 1988; **20**: 233–4.
21 Emanuel EJ, Emanuel LL. Is our AIDS policy ethical? (editorial). *Am J Med* 1987; **83**: 519–20.
22 Henry K, Crossley K. Condoms and the prevention of AIDS (letter). *JAMA* 1986; **256**: 1442.
23 Myers T, Godin G, Calzavara L, Lambert J, Locker D. *The Canadian survey of gay and bisexual men and HIV infection.* Ottawa: Canadian AIDS Society, 1993.
24 Saxton P, Worth H, Hughes T *et al. Male Call: Waea mai tane ma.* Report 7: Gay Community Involvement. Auckland: New Zealand AIDS Foundation, 1998.
25 Tovey SJ, Bonell CP. Condoms: a wider range needed. *BMJ* 1993; **307**: 987.
26 Richters J, Gerofi J, Donovan B. Why do condoms break or slip off in use? An exploratory study. *Int J STD AIDS* 1995; **6**: 11–18.
27 Ross MW. Problems associated with condom use in homosexual men (letter). *Am J Public Health* 1987; **77**: 877.
28 Wigersma L, Oud R. Safety and acceptability of condoms for use by homosexual men as a prophylactic against transmission of HIV during anogenital sexual intercourse. *BMJ* 1987; **295**: 94.
29 Karlsmark T, Segest E, Grindsted J, Bay H. AIDS prevention: free condoms from an STD clinic in Copenhagen (letter). *Genitourin Med* 1989; **65**: 196–202.
30 Sheeran P, Abraham C. Measurement of condom use in 72 studies of HIV-prevention behaviour: a critical review. *Patient Educ Counsel* 1994; **24**: 199–216.
31 Steiner M, Trussell J, Glover L, Joanis C, Spruyt A, Dorflinger L. Standardized protocols for condom breakage and slippage trials: a proposal. *Am J Public Health* 1994; **84**: 1897–900.
32 van Griensven GJP, de Vroome EMM, Tielman RAP, Coutinho RA. Failure rate of condoms during anogenital intercourse in homosexual men. *Genitourin Med* 1988; **64**: 344–6.
33 Tindall B, Swanson C, Donovan B, Cooper DA. Sexual practices and condom usage in a cohort of homosexual men in relation to human immunodeficiency virus status. *Med J Aust* 1989; **151**: 318–22.
34 Thompson JL, Yager TJ, Martin JL. Estimated condom failure and frequency of condom use among gay men. *Am J Public Health* 1993; **83**: 1409–13.
35 Richters J, Donovan B, Gerofi J, Watson L. Low condom breakage rate in commercial sex (letter). *Lancet* 1988; **2**: 1487–8.
36 Golombok S, Sketchley J, Rust J. Condom failure among homosexual men. *J Acquir Immune Defic Syndr* 1989; **2**: 404–9.
37 Richters J, Donovan B, Gerofi J. How often do condoms break or slip off in use? *Int J STD AIDS* 1993; **4**: 90–4.
38 Sparrow MJ, Lavill K. Breakage and slippage of condoms in family planning clients. *Contraception* 1994; **50**: 117–29.
39 Weinstock HS, Lindan C, Bolan G, Kegeles SM, Hearst N. Factors associated with condom use in a high-risk heterosexual population. *Sex Transm Dis* 1993; **20**: 14–20.
40 Golombok S, Sheldon J. Evaluation of a thicker condom for use as a prophylactic against HIV transmission. *AIDS Educ Prev* 1994; **6**: 454–8.
41 Benton KWK, Jolley D, Smith AMA, Gerofi J, Moodie R. An actual use comparison of condoms meeting Australian and Swiss standards: results of a double-blind crossover trial. *Int J STD AIDS* 1997; **8**: 427–31.
41 Grady WR, Tanfer K. Condom breakage and slippage among men in the United States. *Fam Plann Perspect* 1994; **26**: 107–12.

42 Steiner M, Piedrahita C, Glover L, Joanis C. Can condom users likely to experience failure be identified? *Fam Plann Perspect* 1993; **25**: 220–6.

43 Saracco A, Musicco M, Nicolosi A *et al.* Man-to-woman sexual transmission of HIV: longitudinal study of 343 steady partners of infected men. *J Acquir Immune Defic Syndr* 1993; **6**: 497–502.

44 Deschamps MM, Pape JW, Hafner A, Johnson WD Jr. Heterosexual transmission of HIV in Haiti. *Ann Intern Med* 1996; **125**: 324–30.

45 Smith AMA, Jolley D, Hocking J, Benton K, Gerofi J. Does additional lubricant affect condom slippage and breakage? *Int J STD AIDS* 1998; **9**: 330–5.

46 Voeller B, Coulson AH, Bernstein GS, Nakamura RM. Mineral oil lubricants cause rapid deterioration of latex condoms. *Contraception* 1989; **39**: 95–102.

47 Voeller B. Persistent condom breakage (poster). *The scientific and social challenge: V International Conference on AIDS, Montréal, Québec, Canada, June 4–9, 1989.* Abstract W.A.P.99.

48 Smith AMA, Jolley D, Hocking J, Benton K, Gerofi J. Does penis size influence condom slippage and breakage? *Int J STD AIDS* 1998; **9**: 444–7.

49 Smith AMA, Jolley D, Hocking J, Benton K, Gerofi J. Factors affecting men's liking of condoms they have used. *Int J STD AIDS.* 1999; **10**: 258–62.

50 Silverman BG, Gross TP. Use and effectiveness of condoms during anal intercourse: a review. *Sex Transm Dis* 1996; **24**: 11–17.

51 Free MJ, Skiens EW, Morrow MM. Relationship between condom strength and failure during use. *Contraception,* 1980; **22**: 31–7.

52 Gerofi J, Shelley G, Donovan B. A study of the relationship between tensile testing of condoms and breakage in use. *Contraception* 1991; **43**(2): 177–85.

53 Russell-Brown P, Piedrahita C, Foldesy R, Steiner M, Townsend J. Comparison of condom breakage during human use with performance in laboratory testing. *Contraception* 1992; **45**: 429–37.

54 Steiner M, Foldesy R, Cole D, Carter E. Study to determine the correlation between condom breakage in human use and laboratory test results. *Contraception*; **46**: 279–88.

55 Santana H, Richters J. *Sites of sexual activity among men: sex-on-premises venues in Sydney.* Research monograph 5. Sydney: National Centre in HIV Social Research, 1998.

10 Social marketing of condoms

PHILIP D HARVEY

Social marketing consists in the use of expertise and resources from the commercial sector to achieve objectives in the "social" sector. More specifically, social marketing relies on commercial marketing resources – the physical infrastructure of the commercial distribution system, especially distributors, wholesalers, and retailers, and the profit motive of those who participate in these commercially based systems, to achieve a social objective.

Thus, the social marketing of condoms calls for:

- the warehousing and transport of condoms by a distribution agent, working through wholesalers or directly to shops and stores
- the storage and over-the-counter sale of condoms by many thousands of retailers, and
- mass-media advertising of the (branded) condoms, plus other forms of sales promotion.

The latter have included everything from sporting event sponsorship to mobile film units (showing movies with interspersed contraceptive ads), to brand advertising on boat sails, shopping bags, T-shirts, baseball caps, key chains, and similar means (see Figure 10.1).

Part of the magic of the system lies in the fact that the physical infrastructure and its profit-motivated personnel are already in place, and need not be created or specially trained. Commercial retailers and wholesalers in developing countries have shown that they are more than willing to add condoms to their line, especially

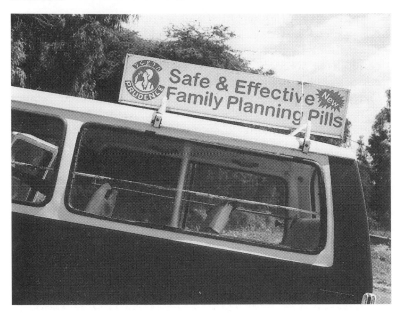

Figure 10.1   These signs atop taxi vans, promoting Prudence oral contraceptives, are a completely new advertising medium in Ethiopia, and they attract a lot of attention.

when they see that these attractively packaged, subsidised contraceptives move quickly off their shelves when supported by mass-media advertising.

Social marketing has turned out to be a nearly ideal way of making condoms widely available to people who want and need them throughout the world. In 1997, nearly a billion condoms (937 million) were sold to more than 16 million couples in 60 social marketing programmes in 55 countries.

Condoms and social marketing have worked together well for the following reasons.

- Condoms are not restricted to any particular type of retail outlet. In almost all countries, they may be made legally available not only in pharmacies and chemist shops, but also in: food stores, kiosks, supermarkets, barbershops; in the tiniest little shops sometimes selling only condoms, cigarettes, and matches; and in the many retail outlets that may be associated with high-risk sexual activity, such as bars, nightclubs, hotels and motels, and inside brothels.

- Condoms are price sensitive and often an impulse purchase, sometimes bought one or two at a time. Social marketing can take full advantage of this because social marketers can price condoms at precisely that level where the largest possible number of people can afford them. Even then, the price can still be high enough to keep the profit-oriented interest of the retailer fully engaged, and to impart a quality image to the product.
- Condoms have a long shelf-life, normally upwards of three years. This means that, even when demand may be low in a particular area or a particular shop, retailers can keep them on hand without fear of imminent spoilage.
- Condoms are amenable to branding and to brand advertising. There are hundreds of brands of condoms in contraceptive social marketing (CSM) programmes around the world; brands meaning "protection", "shield", "life", "trust", "prudence", as well as the names of animals, like *Panther* and *Bull*. There are also names that mean nothing at all, like the commercial brand *Durex*. But branding works with condoms particularly well. One reason is that people everywhere are still embarrassed to ask for condoms, and brand names, when heavily promoted, often become generic, thus making the product easier to ask for, see Figure 10.2.

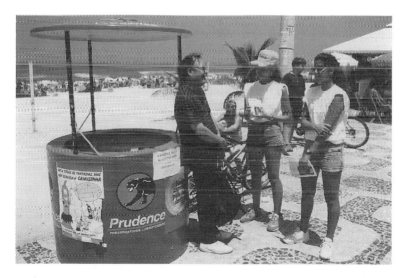

Figure 10.2 Prudence condoms, sold through the social marketing programme in Brazil, are promoted by well-tanned field educators on the beaches during carnival and other festivals.

149

Pricing

When condom social marketing got underway three decades ago, it was widely believed that there would be some conflict between pricing for maximum sales (pricing low) and pricing for maximum incentive to the trade (pricing medium, or even high). The tension never developed. Social marketing managers have found that they can charge a significant price when selling to the trade and still meet the "one per cent" standard for pricing condoms to the consumer. The one per cent standard refers to the fact that a year's supply of contraceptives should cost no more than 1 per cent of annual per-capita GNP. For condoms, which are more price sensitive than other contraceptives, my own research suggests that 100 condoms (an average year's supply), should cost no more than 0.7 per cent of per-capita GNP or, alternatively, 0.25 per cent of purchasing power parity (PPP)-adjusted income. Thus in a country of US$300 per capita GNP and US$1 200 PPP-adjusted income (in a typical low-income country the PPP figure is roughly four times per-capita GNP), 100 condoms should cost the consumer no more than US$3 and, ideally, no more than US$2.10 (0.7 per cent of per-capita GNP). For a fuller discussion of social marketing pricing, see Ciszewski and Harvey (1995)[1] and Harvey (1994).[2]

With this requirement it might be supposed that trade margins would be so thin as to make socially marketed condoms unattractive to retailers and others in the trade distribution chain. If US$300 were a typical per-capita GNP for a low-income developing country (it is), and we could charge the consumer only US$2.10 for 100 condoms, or just 2 cents per condom, it might seem that there is little left for the trade. Should the first tier of trade pay the project 1 cent per condom, mark up 35 per cent, and another middleman marks up 15 per cent, the retailer could mark up 30 per cent from there to reach the 2 cent final price. But while 30 per cent is a healthy margin, it amounts to less than 0.5 cents per condom. That is just 1.4 cents per three-pack to the retailer, or about 32 cents in margin for a half-gross box, a quantity that might take two or three weeks for a typical shopkeeper to sell.

The reason this works is that 1.4 cents means a lot more to the retailer in a very low-income country than in a wealthier country. That 32 cents per half-gross box might, for example, represent a whole day's wage for a labourer in Bangladesh or Ethiopia and it can therefore represent a significant source of income to a small shopkeeper.

Another reason that this subsidised arrangement works is that shopkeepers recognise that a low priced product will likely be a very fast-moving product. This is particularly true if the product is backed by substantial mass-media advertising, as socially marketed condoms almost always are. Indeed the advertising budgets deployed in support of socially marketed condoms usually exceed, by quite a lot, the amount of advertising that could be profitably employed if the condoms were selling for full commercial rates, even high commercial rates. In DKT International's Ethiopia project, for example, advertising and promotion expenditures in 1997 were 300 per cent of primary sales (sales to the first tier of trade). Obviously, no commercial producer could live with such a ratio. Social marketers can do it because donor funding foots most of the bill.

As the number of condom social marketing projects proliferated in the 1980s and 90s, I expected we would see at least a few projects selling to the trade for nominal amounts, receiving essentially nothing in the way of sales income, in order to meet the consumer pricing guidelines. It has not happened: for one thing, maximising consumer demand requires that condoms not be priced *too* low. If a product seems unbelievably cheap, consumers question its quality, especially if it is seen as coming from the government. For this, and perhaps other, reasons, the 1 per cent standard has been met in a large number of programmes and still the projects sell to the trade for something like half the final consumer price, providing at least some income to the programme.

Social marketing in socialist economies

Interestingly, the social marketing of contraceptives in communist, formerly communist, or otherwise socialist economic settings appears to be no more difficult than in more free-market economies. There are trade-offs: family planning tends to be widely understood in communist countries, for example. For whatever reasons, developing countries like Vietnam and China have long promoted birth control, and the concept is widely understood. Furthermore, while governments can be relatively effective at promoting propaganda, they are notoriously bad at providing attractively packaged consumer goods. We have found in Vietnam, for example, that there is an especially strong demand for nicely packaged contraceptives that are, and appear to be, of high quality. Such goods are never provided by governments.

Offsetting this is the tendency of socialist governmentts to think they can do everything. In China, it has been difficult to break the government monopoly on the sale of contraceptives, though it is proving to be gradually possible. In Vietnam, our demonstration of the effectiveness of the social marketing of contraceptives led the government to go into the social marketing business itself, simultaneously withdrawing its material support to the DKT programme. Until that time DKT International received substantial quantities of condoms supplied by the government. Such problems, however, are no greater than those we face in more traditional, free-market economies like the Philippines and Malaysia, where family planning is less widely understood and less readily accepted.

India represents an interesting combination. The government has traditionally leaned toward socialism, and has long operated its own contraceptive social marketing programme. Over the current decade, however, the government has increasingly privatised the project (as well as much else in the economy), now supplying very large quantities of government-subsidised contraceptives to four private social marketing organisations, including two affiliates of DKT. So, while the challenges of social marketing in socialist-oriented economies tend to be different, they seem to be no greater and no less than the challenges facing social marketers elsewhere.

A case study in contrasts: Ethiopia and Brazil

While the differences facing social marketing managers in socialist vs less socialist economies are unpredictable and hard to categorise, the differences between social marketing in poorly developed economies as against operating such programmes in the more advanced developing countries are dramatic and consistent. These differences are well illustrated by DKT International's marketing programmes in Ethiopia and Brazil.

In Ethiopia, the programme functions in one of the lowest income environments in the world. With per-capita GNP of about US$120, the 1 per cent rule tells us that the consumer cost of 100 condoms should not be much over US$1.00; a single condom can cost the buyer only 1 cent or less. With the project's price to the trade about half the consumer price, this means that there can be no thought of recovering the cost of the condoms or even a substantial fraction of that cost. Packaged condoms on the international market cost 3–4 cents each in 1998; in Ethiopia the cost is slightly higher because the donor, USAID, is required to buy American-made condoms. Thus DKT's recovery amounts to less than 20 per cent of the ex-factory price of the product. This is not unusual in condom social marketing, especially in Africa, and well illustrates the social marketer's ironic cliché: "The more we sell the more we lose".

In Brazil, in sharp contrast, the 1 per cent rule permits the project to charge a consumer price of more than 30 cents per condom (per-capita GNP = US$3600). Even with extra duties imposed by the Brazilian government, and extra-high port costs in Santos, the world's most expensive port, the branded cost per packaged condom is about 11 cents after duties have been paid. We can sell to the trade for 13 cents and still maintain an average consumer cost of a little over 30 cents. (The actual price charged by Brazilian retailers varies; decades of hyperinflation have accustomed Brazilian consumers to the fact that costs are likely to fluctuate and that the prices of consumer goods are not printed on packages. Even with inflation under control these practices and expectations persist.) This means that project managers can begin to think about using product sales to cover some operating costs and even, perhaps, reach complete financial sustainability. At a true margin of just 2 cents per condom, sales of 34 million condoms (the 1997 total) means a gross profit of nearly $700,000 – enough to pay salaries, rents, and at least part of the advertising, training, and education costs. Brazil is, in fact, totally different from Ethiopia (and many other countries) because in Brazil, the more we sell the *less* we lose.

The Ethiopian programme is described by DKT's project manager in Addis Ababa, Chris Purdy:

When DKT started in 1990, Ethiopia was just completing a long civil war and exiting from a centralized socialist economy that knew nothing of consumer marketing. On top of that the logistics were and are especially daunting.

Ethiopia is cut up by mountains and deserts and the populations are remote and rural. Towns are separated by long stretches of dusty roads and fields. In between, rural agrarian populations live in small villages and communities where the formal commercial sector is practically non-existent. Rough roads and heavy rainy seasons make it often impossible and always difficult to reach those areas where condoms are needed (see Figure 10.3).

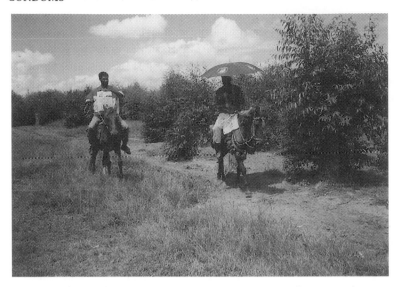

Figure 10.3   Good roads are few and far between in Ethiopia. HIWOT condoms have to be distributed by whatever means are available for crossing fields and traversing dirt tracks.

On the other hand, there are several things that make selling condoms easier. First, we entered into an economy where consumer advertising was virtually non-existent. When DKT entered the marketplace with TV and radio ads, our ads were noticed, read, and usually believed, because there was so little advertising "clutter."

Furthermore the cost of space is very low, because there is so little disposable income in the economy. Even with a small budget, we have been able to advertise heavily, dominating the radio especially. In addition, DKT was among the first marketers to engage in such simple yet (for Ethiopia)revolutionary ideas as the use of signboards on top of taxis and interesting and colorful point-of-purchase materials. In 1998, DKT introduced an oral contraceptive package with a photograph of an Ethiopian woman – the first time in the history of the country that an Ethiopian has been featured on any package for any product.

The result is that the *Hiwot* condom has quickly established a major market presence. Indeed, *Hiwot* has become the generic term for condom in Ethiopia, with an estimated 99 per cent market share. The term "Hiwot" is so thoroughly associated with condoms that I have had women complain to me that they were named *Hiwot* (a common female name meaning "Life") and wished they could change their names. This could not have happened in a more advanced economy on a media budget of only $300–400 000 per year, but here that's enough to revolutionize the role and image of condoms nationwide.

On the negative side for our marketing effort is the fact that 85 per cent of the population lives a long way from the nearest paved road, and there are few real stores in the remote rural areas. So our salesmen and women have to drive the 45 kilometers, for example, through a non-road terrain, to sell one or two boxes of condoms. This makes for slow, expensive sales.

In Ethiopia, DKT is pretty much the only game in town if we speak of HIV prevention on a national level. For a country with 2.6 million infected people, the Ethiopian Government response has been very weak. Much of the burden seems to be on DKT to provide whatever gets provided in the way of information and condoms. Knowledge, of course, does not always translate into condom use, and anecdotal evidence suggests that many Ethiopian men feel that the use of a condom prevents ejaculation (not pleasurable) and would rather find a virgin, young girl, or simply take the risk rather than use a condom.

Thus, in Ethiopia we have a classic case of a very poor country where the social marketing programme is contributing a very substantial portion of all of the family planning and HIV prevention available to the population. To reach large numbers (DKT's programme sold 28 million condoms in Ethiopia in 1997), the product must be priced way below its factory cost. The idea of generating revenue by selling more condoms is, for the time being at least, not a consideration.

The role of the condom social marketing project in Brazil – with per-capita GNP more than 30 times Ethiopia's – has been dramatically different. There were two major condom manufacturers in Brazil when DKT International first arrived. The role of the project has been to shake up the oligopoly enjoyed by those two companies, to make it possible for those companies as well as others to import lower-priced condoms, and to introduce serious price competition for the first time, thus lowering the price of condoms to all Brazilians and dramatically increasing the total condom market.

Carlos Ferreros, DKT's manager in São Paulo, describes the Brazilian programme:

Prior to the introduction of DKT's *Prudence* condom in 1991, the Brazilian condom market was around 50 million units a year, with prices per condom ranging from US$0.70 to $1.00. Condoms were not promoted and marketers were content with constant volume as it required little or no expense to support existing market shares. The market at the time was dominated by two major brands, *Jontex* and *Olla*, both of which were traditional brands, having been in existence for around 20 years. Another player was *Blowtex* with a minor share. These three brands were produced locally and virtually no imports were allowed.

This changed in the early 1990s when Brazil officially opened its market to imports. DKT International was invited by the state government to establish a social marketing program in São Paulo and took advantage of the market opening. We imported condoms, creating our own brand, *Prudence,* and proceeded to aggressively market it at a consumer price of $0.17 to $0.20. Other trading companies took note and proceeded to import their own brands, pricing them somewhere between *Prudence* and *Jontex.* A pricing revolution was underway.

At the same time, the incidence of HIV transmission and the number of AIDS cases rose dramatically, and the government began to expand AIDS information programs. This was augmented by efforts by non-governmental organizations (NGOs) to increase awareness and prevention programs among their own constituents.

Condoms are not traditionally advertised via electronic media in Brazil, which in any case are very expensive. Our efforts could not, because of cost, utilize television or print media. A 30–second spot with 3 million viewers might cost $200 in Ethiopia; in Brazil a comparable price-tag is $15 000. DKT therefore opted to make its brand known to at-risk low-income populations (its primary target group) by developing a support network among a number of NGOs. This entailed either selling at a very preferential price, or giving out samples to these NGOs, and supplying them with *Prudence*-oriented educational and promotional material.

DKT sponsors NGOs that have year-round programs to educate target populations, and supplies these NGOs with the wherewithal to help offset expenses. For example, DKT supplies APTA-BARONG with condoms that this organization can sell as it sets up in various beaches or parks throughout São Paulo state promoting AIDS prevention. This NGO operates out of a mobile trailer on which is mounted a two-meter inflatable condom (see Figure 10.4). Revenue generated is used to help offset expenses.

We also rely on event marketing. Owing to limited resources, *Prudence* could not engage in Coca-Cola-like exclusive sponsorship of events such as the Olympics. Instead *Prudence* condoms became the sponsor of selected events in crowded beach areas at Carnival, Winterfest, various state and city fairs, etc. (see Figure 10.5). This kind of targeted sponsorship allows the social marketers to affordably operate within the site of the event such as the Rio beaches during Carnival. In a typical event, Prudence kiosks are set up where promoters fan out to distribute educational material and entice revelers to purchase low-priced condoms from the kiosks. These activities often get free coverage on TV and in print.

All of the above (social marketing, government campaigns, NGO activities, increase in imports and competition) have led to a five-fold increase in the Brazilian condom market from 50 million in 1991 to around 250 million in 1997. Significantly, competitive efforts have increased with vigorous trade promotions leading to a lowering of average pricing to around $0.57 per condom in 1997. Where there were three major brands in 1991, there are now eight, plus several minor brands.

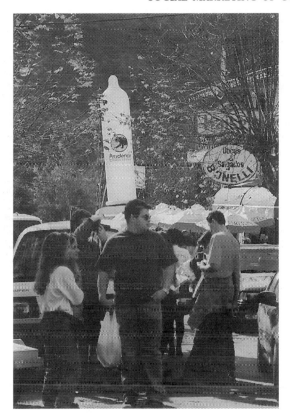

Figure 10.4   This 2m high Prudence condom on the roof of the DKT sales van in Brazil draws crowds who learn about condoms and get free samples.

In 1998, average condom pricing was lowered even further to around $0.48 per condom (the consumer price for *Prudence* was $0.35 in 1998). This was a result of the individual states agreeing to temporarily suspend a VAT-like tax on condoms which averaged around 18 per cent of the suggested consumer price. Early indications are that this led to an increase of around 15 per cent in condom sales.

This temporary lowering of condom taxes was the result of the efforts of the Associação Saude da Familia (ASF), an NGO dedicated to AIDS prevention which took up advocacy as one of its strategies. Studies were presented to the individual state inland revenue departments showing that a lowering of condom taxes would lead to lower prices and higher prevention rates, thus saving the government's resources in long-term health expenditures. Further efforts by the ASF are being directed to declare condoms a "basic commodity" to ensure that these taxes are permanently lifted.

157

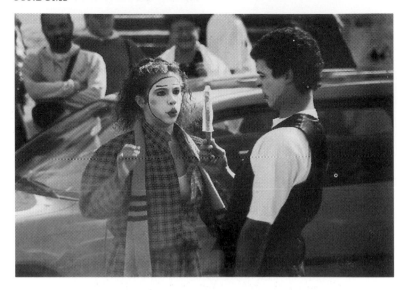

Figure 10.5 Street theatre in Brazil promotes condom use and gets people laughing about an otherwise embarassing product.

Discussion

Pricing is the cornerstone of contraceptive social marketing, especially for condoms which are more price sensitive than other contraceptive products. Condoms should normally be priced so that 100 condoms cost the consumer around 0.7 per cent of per-capita GNP. It is possible to do this and still produce at least some income to the project though, in low-income countries like Ethiopia, that income stream may be only a fraction of the cost of the contraceptives themselves.

As seen in the dramatic contrast between the social marketing of condoms in Ethiopia and Brazil, the financial structuring of CSM programmes can vary dramatically. In poor countries the rule must be: "The more we sell the more we lose". Our purpose is primarily humanitarian not financial. But when per capita GNP exceeds $2500, it becomes possible to begin recovering some programme costs from the gross margin generated by the difference between the CIF cost of condoms and the (slightly higher) selling price of the product to the first tier of the trade. Then we can begin to significantly reduce donor contributions to the programme.

Social marketing programmes are supplying condoms to more

than 16 million couples around the world, making this perhaps the most significant mode of delivery for subsidised condoms. However, this is only a fraction of what could be done. With millions of new HIV infections every year – most of which will likely be prevented *only* through increased condom use – and a huge unmet demand for condoms for pregnancy prevention, at least three times the present number of couples could be reached through the social marketing mechanism. Increased donor support for social marketing in poor countries, combined with more efficient management and, in the wealthier developing nations, increasing cost recovery, could accomplish this in a relatively short time. Social marketing programmes can be started quickly and expanded efficiently when adequate funding is available.

Further reading

1 Ciszewski RL, Harvey PD. Contraceptive price changes: the impact on sales in Bangladesh. *Internat Fam Plann Perspect* 1995; **21**(4): 150–54.
2 Harvey PD. The impact of prices on condom sales in social marketing programs, 1994. *Stud Fam Plann*; **25**(1): 52–8.

11 Condom availability: barriers to access, barriers to use

WILLIAM P SCHELLSTEDE, MADALINE P
FEINBERG, GINA DALLABETTA

Each year approximately 8 to 10 billion condoms are used, but an estimated 15 billion condoms per year are needed to protect adequately against STD/HIV/AIDS.[1] Although the male latex condom, when used corectly and consistently, is highly effective at both reducing unintended pregnancy and preventing STD/HIV, condom use rates vary considerably around the globe. In developed countries, there is broad access to affordable condoms, although it might be argued that in many communities a certain reticence towards condoms constrains their use. In developing countries, however, regular condom use is low for a number of reasons, among which accessibility is often a major factor, leaving much of the world's population with a limited ability to protect themselves from pregnancy or STD.

Condom use varies greatly between cultures, among subpopulations, and even within high-risk groups. At the same time, numerous studies in a wide variety of settings have found that men report condom use at last intercourse more frequently than do women, and that married men are more likely to use condoms with commercial sex workers (CSWs) or in sexual relationships outside of marriage, than they are with their wives. Similarly, more men than women say they have ever used condoms, have ever heard of condoms, understand that condoms can prevent HIV transmission, or know the closest location where they can obtain condoms. Yet the proportion of men using condoms regularly remains low: despite the HIV/AIDS epidemic and the attention it has focused on using condoms to reduce personal risk, beginning to use condoms is only the third or fourth most common behaviour change among married men, and one of the last behaviour changes identified by married women. Unmarried men and women are more likely to reduce their risk of infection by abstaining from sex or delaying sexual initiation.[1] Further data on condom use/trends is available.[2–7]

Condom availability

The availability of condoms is a measure of the degree to which access to condoms permits them to be considered a viable option for those who would use them to prevent infection or unwanted pregnancy. Preciseness of definition as to whether condoms are effectively available is difficult, however, in many instances, since the involvement of the prospective user is paramount in actually acquiring the condom. For example, a government STD clinic located in a high risk area of a city might supply condoms without charge to those perceiving themselves at risk of infection; if the clinic's hours were 9:00 to 17:00, and if patrons arrived in the area and negotiated their high risk sex mostly late at night, to what degree may one say that the STD clinic's condoms are "available" to them? Even more problematic for purposes of definition is the issue of distance: it might be thought unreasonable to expect villagers to travel 20 miles into the city in order to access condoms; but at what point is proximity no longer an issue? Price can also act as an effective barrier to condom use among the poor where the primary source of condoms is the commercial sector. Finally, are condoms in any practical sense actually available when they are not openly displayed and their use publicly encouraged?

Aware of these conceptual difficulties, the United Nations nevertheless estimates that two-thirds of the world's population has ready and easy access to condoms, where "ready and easy access" denotes that people must spend an average of no more than two hours obtaining supplies and services each month, and spend no more than 1 per cent of their monthly income on condoms.[1] The definition, while perhaps useful in permitting estimates of condom needs on a gross level, presents problems when two different countries are considered, one in which condoms are aggressively promoted, and another in which they are distributed but barely mentioned in public. In the second country, the parameters of the definition may overstate their availability by a wide margin.

161

Condom acceptability and accessibility both influence, and are influenced by, condom availability, which is one explanation why condom use remains low in developing countries. Mehryar's definition of condom accessibility illustrates this complicated interrelationship: "Effective access to condoms [means] . . . A person must have heard of condoms, must be aware of a supply source and must live (or work) within 30 minutes of it".[2] As above, this definition remains less than ideal, if what the person has heard of condoms is mostly negative.

Despite these conceptual difficulties in defining availability, it can be safely said that availability of condoms varies greatly around the world, and that the factors leading to lower levels of availability than would be desired vary greatly, as well. One means of analysing availability is to consider it at the several points of possible intervention, or, namely, at the international, national public and private sectors, and in social marketing.

International availability

It does not appear that the world's condom industry at present is overwhelmed by demand. Indeed, donors currently have considerable latitude in choosing suppliers, and prices have remained relatively stable for the past ten years. If there has been a substantial increase in demand for thin latex film products arising from the AIDS epidemic, it is more for rubber gloves than for condoms. A good deal of the concern about condom supply on a global level comes from interpolating from numbers of people theoretically "at risk" to the numbers of condoms thought needed to protect them. But such large numbers do not represent effective demand, either now or any time in the foreseeable future. The fact is that not every person at risk will use condoms. In Japan and the United States, where purchasing power is for the most part adequate and where it can be assumed that reasonable efforts are made, both to encourage condom use and to make them conveniently available, condom use has not exceeded roughly two to four condoms per capita. If that is a safe upper limit for condom use, then supplying the world's condom needs, certainly over the near term, is well within the limits of the industry's capabilities.

On the other hand, it can be said that condom supplies are not adquate for programmes meant to address the very poor. It is not the case that the industry is unable to produce condoms in adequate quantities – indeed, there is every reason to believe that condom production could increase substantially over time, given the appropriate levels of demand – but rather that international programmes do not have ready access to condom supplies through international donors.

Beginning in the mid-1970s the United States Agency for International Development (USAID) took on the major role of supplying contraceptives, including condoms, to developing country programmes. In retrospect it can be said that such programmes have, in aggregate, been enormously successful: the world's population growth rate is down, and most developing countries, particularly in Asia and Latin America, have viable growing family planning programmes. However, and perhaps ironically, it is this very success that has constrained the ability or the willingness of donors, including USAID, to meet the AIDS epidemic with liberal supplies of condoms. A growing proportion of resources available to USAID was being consumed in contraceptive supply, and its other activities relating to the design, management and evaluation of population programming, activities critical to efficient and ethical programmes, became more difficult to support. Eventually, commodity procurement and shipment were reduced in budget. In the late 1980s USAID was purchasing nearly one billion condoms per year; current levels are less than one-half that. In part because control over a larger portion of USAID's budget has been shifted to the field, but also because of generally lower levels of funding overall, USAID's recent, large AIDS prevention programmes have not had direct access to condom supplies. Other donors, notably the European Community and the German government, have recently become more active in supplying condoms, but this involvement is limited to a few countries, such as Bangladesh and Pakistan, and has not yet become global in its effect.

The result of this more difficult supply situation is that condom programming – and therefore condom availability – has in many instances been constrained. For example, USAID declined to supply condoms to the condom social marketing component of the AIDS prevention programme it was supporting in Brazil. As a result, the social marketing project had to price its condoms at a level that permitted the purchase of replacement stocks.

Overall, social marketing had a significant impact on condom availability in Brazil, largely by introducing aggressive advertising and lower prices than commercial distributors had been accustomed to, and by fighting to reduce taxes and import restrictions. The result has been a remarkable increase in the brands available in the market, more lively competition among local manufacturers, and a tripling of the commercial market for condoms. On the other hand, had the social marketers been able to price their brand at a substantially lower level, condom availability to the very poor would have been enhanced to a more significant degree than it has been.

National availability: public sector

As suggested in the opening paragraphs of this chapter, condom programming that does not take into account the circumstances of the target of such programming may be limited in the extent to which it effectively makes condoms "available". National programmes that expend efforts to distribute condoms through their public health and family planning service delivery systems may be only partly successful. Supplying condoms through the public sector is probably a necessary step, especially if the physical distribution is accompanied by a carefully designed and aggressive effort to encourage their proper and regular use. Indeed, some types of public sector facilities, such as STD clinics, have contact with populations at extremely high risk of infection, and the opportunity to reach these individuals with good information and encouragement about condoms and to provide them at least with samples cannot be missed.

On the other hand, quite apart from the financial challenge of procuring large quantities of condoms, the constraints inherent to the public sector must be recognised. First, the public sector systems are most often already overwhelmed by the demands made upon them. At the national level, logistics capabilities face generally severe limitations, and placing a new, large volume commodity like condoms in the system frequently leads to inefficiencies, leakage, stock-outs and spoilage.

The logistics difficulties found in the public sector can be addressed. Indeed, the effect of USAID's investments in the management of contraceptive supply over the past 20 years has had a profound effect in many countries. However, condom programming is being done within the public health structure, and often the improvements made in the logistics of family planning do not extend to most health facilities. When condom supplies enter the systems that customarily handle drugs and other health-related commodities, problems do arise. They are often fundamental problems, not readily amenable to easy or quick solution.

As suggested above, there are limitations to the suitability of the service delivery points as vehicles for efficient condom delivery. Most significant is the extent of duties and responsibilities other-wise present, particularly in health posts, where handling condom supplies will most often assume a very low staff priority. Even in family planning clinics, condoms are widely and mistakenly thought to have a low efficacy, and, even when condom use is not actively discouraged, they are seldom promoted with real enthusiasm by family planning workers. Moreover, they are an extremely simple method, and while they do require the users to acquire some level of competence in their use, they require little intellectual involvement of the providers compared with other methods. Finally, family planning facilities serve a relatively small portion of the population, a portion that, in most societies, are not at the highest risk of HIV infection.

In short, public sector service delivery points seldom achieve significant levels of condom distribution, either in terms of volume or of epidemiological targeting. Put another way, the availability of condoms in clinics and health posts, while highly desirable, does not often equate to widespread availability to the population as a whole, nor to effective protection of those most seriously at risk.

Some public sector programmes attempt to overcome distribu-tion constraints on health and family planning facilities by engaging outreach workers. While this extension can increase distribution significantly, it is expensive, not only in the cost of the workers themselves, but also for the management and super-visory apparatus that must accompany it.

National availability: private sector

In the industrialised world, virtually all condoms are distribu-ted through the retail system. This distribution is generally though adquate and cost efficient. Little "unmet demand" is perceived in Europe, North America, or the Far East, and, apart from a few exceptions (e.g. the military, prisons), there seems little reason to recommend intervention from the public health community.

On the other hand, left entirely to commercial firms, the con-dom industry has not been notable for its boldness in legitimising condom use and bringing condoms into the mainstream of social acceptability. In the United States, condoms (and other contraceptives) have in the past two decades become more visible in retail outlets, but it must be noted that a non-profit organisation fought in the Supreme Court and succeeded in overturning laws prohibiting their display (PSI vs. Cary, *et al.*, 1976).

Indeed, in *The Condom Industry in the United States* James S Murphy[8] argues persuasively that condom manufacturers in the USA constitute an oligarchy, and have not actively pursued massive increases in sales, largely as a matter of strategy, preferring to protect the stability of their markets to the rough and tumble of competition. Barriers to advertising were seldom challenged; only recently campaigns addressing the AIDS epidemic financed by the US Centers for Disease Control began to break new ground, and condom advertisements followed suit, though seldom outside men's magazines.

In the developing world, with few exeptions, condoms are not easily found in the private sector, and almost never outside large cities, and then only in small numbers. Most of this absence can be explained by the modest purchasing power to be found there: people by definition are mostly very poor. But a large part of the explanation can also be found in the attitudes of the private sector toward products such as condoms. Even pharmaceutical companies with hormonal contraceptives to sell, seldom took on the battles required to market them aggressively in poor countries, characterised most often by religious conservatism and pronatalist mores. Contraceptives seldom make up a major part of a pharmaceutical company's income; compared with antacids and analgesics they are only minor, and certainly not worth alienating the government in battling over restrictions on their sale and distribution. With condoms, not only would the marketers have to overcome all the acceptability problems faced elsewhere, they would also have to take on the religious governmental establishments, as well.

Social marketing

Virtually all condom distribution in the developing world that has reached public health or demographic significance has come from "social marketing". First fielded in India in the late 1960s with the sale of a government-owned condom brand, Nirodh, social marketing in this context denotes the marketing of a subsidised product believed by its sponsors to have an important social value when purchased and used by the public. Supported now by a number of international donors, USAID first recognised the potential of social marketing for increasing the availability of contraceptives massively by putting contraceptives into a system that already operates with remarkable efficiency and that brings to the doorsteps virtually all the goods that are used in everyday life, by everbody, the wealthy and the poor, the rural and the urban. The urban slums and the isolated villages are all served by the commercial retail system.

Compared with public sector distribution, social marketing can achieve remarkable cost savings to the government or donor by shifting the cost of distribution to the user: in the early model of social marketing, contraceptives were brought into a country and sold to a wholesaler at a cost that did not cover the cost of the product, but helped defray some or all of the cost of promotion. The wholesaler sold to lower level distributors who, in turn, sold to retailers. The expenses of the wholesaler, distributors, and retailers (and their incentives, or profits) were all subsumed in the retail price charged the customer. If considerable product volume is involved, that retail price can be modest, indeed: for example, in Bangladesh in the early 1980s, a condom was sold to the consumer for less than US$0.01; volume passed 100 million condoms within 6 years of launch.

Later models of social marketing do not assume a "free" supply of product (for reasons described above in relation to international donors), and retail prices have been higher. Still, the fundamental elements for massively increasing the availability of condoms remain: first, a core of marketing experts whose motivation is not the maximising of income but enhancing access to quality condoms; second, sufficient funding to advertise and promote a branded product; third, the demographic and/or epidemiological input required to target sales to the appropriate populations; and fourth, a tie into the national distribution system used by commercial traders, based on a ladder of margins on the retail price that provides each step with a fair and adequate incentive to be part of the effort.

Recent social marketing to reduce the risk of HIV infection (largely financed by USAID) has produced dramatic increases in condom distribution in a number of countries, including Brazil, Tanzania, Nigeria, Ethiopia, Haiti, and South Africa. Not only has the total number of condoms increased significantly on a national level, in most instances successful efforts have been

167

made to target sales to high risk populations. For example, in Haiti the social marketers helped non-governmental organisations (NGOs) to begin retailing condoms to their own clients and members; NGO sales came to represent one-third of total sales. In Cameroon, Ethiopia and elsewhere, prostitutes were recruited and trained to become peer educators and condom retailers. In Brazil, where there were philosophical and legal barriers to NGOs becoming involved in retail trade, special "promotoras", or sales women, were paid to ensure that condom stocks were adequate at bars, hotels and bordellos where the NGOs were active.

It must be emphasised that these latter activities are not likely to be undertaken by a commercial firm in the normal course of business. Sales to NGOs, or peer educators, and stocking low-volume outlets such as bars, would be considered expensive distractions by a firm intent on making profit. Indeed such activities, key to reaching those most in need of ready access to condoms, are the principal "social" component of condom social marketing in the era of the AIDS epidemic.

At the same time, a larger market for the condoms is also aggressively pursued. High sales volume is desirable in social marketing, in part to generate income to finance further promotion and to lessen the management costs to the sponsors, and in part to promote condoms as contraceptives. But successful sales to the general population are also important, even critical, to the success of the sales targeted to those at high risk of infection, because they reflect a wider, more generalised acceptance of condom use at the level of social norms. Donors in AIDS prevention, in their understandable need to be efficient, have sometimes argued for social marketing programmes limited to those targeted sales; sales to the general public seem less efficient in that they are used in less risky situations: they prevent relatively few infections for a given number of condoms. But a condom distribution and promotion programme that attempted to limit its sales to those at high risk would, in effect, be asking its market to identify itself as marginal to society. The degree to which these people are marginalised by many societies make this request unreasonable.

It should be said that social marketing has proved its effectiveness in a wide variety of settings. Success has been seen in Catholic, Protestant and Islamic countries. Even in a country where communism still provides the basic economic tenets, free market reforms in Vietnam in recent years have permitted social marketing, and between 1994 and 1998, private sector sales of condoms rose from 17 to 51 per cent. Social marketing has operated there in virtually the same manner as elsewhere: over this period condoms became more publicly visible, ultimately increasing knowledge of condoms and encouragement for their use; and consumers there, as elsewhere, have responded postively to their being more conveniently available, and being able to purchase them in relative anonymity.[9]

Condom acceptability and accessibility

Just as long distances and high condom prices can make condoms inaccessible, social and political norms governing condom use and sexuality can make condoms equally inaccessible, even when condoms are physically and economically available. While condoms may be readily available in some areas, religious and cultural beliefs that condoms are unacceptable can all but proscribe their actual purchase and use. Even in areas where condoms are considered available in developing countries, usually the more urban areas, condom use in most countries is relatively low.

Studies of condom use and sexual behaviour [2,4–7] have documented that high levels of AIDS awareness and the understanding that condoms can reduce the risk of HIV infection do not necessarily translate into increased condom use. Further, a stated intention or desire to use condoms in the future is not indicative of an increase in actual use.[10] While some subpopulations (such as married women) are unaware of the extent to which their sexual behaviour, or the sexual behaviour of their spouses, put them at risk, even women who understand their risk may still not use condoms. It is this complex of human social, gender, religious and economic relationships that makes condom promotion a challenge, even in the face of AIDS. Condom accessibility, by all definitions, remains the most impotant obstacle to the initiation and continued use condoms by those desiring to prevent pregnancy and prevent the transmission of STIs.

Barriers to condom use

Over the past 15 years the explosive HIV/AIDS epidemic has brought renewed attention to condoms, but only a limited increase in condom use. The use of condoms for disease prevention, now promoted separately from pregnancy prevention,

169

has raised a new set of obstacles to their correct and sustained use.

Programmes encouraging condom use may still be associated with the earlier days of population assistance when condoms were promoted as a method for "population control." Well established fears of developed nations distributing condoms in the hopes of perpetuating an African genocide have more recently shifted to suspicions of developed countries infecting condoms with the AIDS virus or making holes in condoms before distributing them in Africa. Myths of various origins relate the potential dangers of condom use; for example, a belief that condoms can make a woman infertile or may slip off and travel up inside her body. In populations which emphasize the exchange of bodily fluids during sex the ends of condoms may be cut off before use.

One of the strongest complaints against using condoms is that they feel unnatural, uncomfortable, and decrease sexual pleasure and spontaneity.[11] Condom use runs counter to expectations of masculinity and imply a physical vulnerability. Men may also fear perceived side-effects of condom use on their partners.

Early in the AIDS epidemic commercial sex workers (CSWs) were identified as a high risk group and targeted with condom promotion programmes. The outcome of such programmes has been successful in reducing HIV transmission among CSWs and their clients, most remarkably in Thailand, but has also had the effect of closely associating condom use with commercial sex, promiscuity, and sex outside of marriage.[12] In some regions, especially in Africa, it is accepted and often expected that men have sexual relationships outside of marriage.[13] If condoms are used, their use will often be reserved for extra-marital relationships, as sex within marriage is expected to be natural, with no barrier to the exchange of bodily fluids. Although both men and women may understand that they face a risk of disease transmission, to discuss condom use would require acknowledging the existence of extra-marital or regular multiple partners.

Married women in monogamous relationships can be especially exposed to sexual risk due to the behaviour of their husbands. They have limited ability to make decisions about when and whether to have sex and therefore are unable to ensure that condoms are used. Disadvantaged socially and economically, women may face serious repercussions if they insist on condom use with or withhold sex from their partners. Discussing condom use might imply that a woman believes her partner has other sexual partners, or that she herself has other partners. Women who insist on condom use face possible physical harm, divorce or estrangement. It may be easier to face the long-term risk of possible HIV infection than to face the potentially immediate consequences. In either case, women are unable to entirely eliminate their risk of becoming infected. Unmarried women have higher rates of condom use, as they may not be as dependent on a man who is not their husband. Although women are particularly vulnerable, both men and women report having difficulty discussing sex and condom use with their partners. Both fear that by raising the subject they would incriminate themselves or offend their partner(s).

A survey of HIV-positive and HIV-negative women in Uganda[5] found that women are more likely to support condom use in marriage than are men, and that 15 per cent of women would want to use condoms if their husbands found it acceptable. Women in this group reported that their primary method for reducing their risk of HIV/AIDS was to be monogamous, but this strategy will clearly not protect women in the long term.

Where a woman's worth is determined largely by her ability to have children, she is under extreme social pressure to become pregnant. High STD rates worldwide have subsequently led to increasing rates of infertility. In regions where women want to be pregnant, and where becoming pregnant is becoming increasingly difficult due to infertility, AIDS prevention messages promoting condoms have an understandably limited impact. The pressure to have children can be so great that an HIV-positive woman may still want to become pregnant, even when she knows that it is possible to pass HIV on to her child. High infant mortality rates and social pressures to have children can make it less risky for an HIV-positive woman to have children who she knows may be infected, than not to have children at all.[13]

Unmarried youth face all of the same barriers as adults and married couples, and additional barriers due to their age and social expectations about young people and sexuality. Younger people who have been raised with the threat of AIDS are aware of the protection afforded by condoms, and rates of condom use among young males are increasing. In some countries family planning and contraceptive services are only legal for married people, despite the rates, acknowledged or unacknowledged, of sexual activity among youth. Even where condoms are available to youth, clinic staff may make it difficult to access services, or refuse to provide services to them at all. Attendance at local clinics does not offer youth anonymity, and the threat of encountering a relative or acquaintance is enough to discourage them from trying to obtain condoms.

Despite the considerable social and cultural obstacles to condom use, one of the greatest barriers to condom use for both men and women remains an unfamiliarity with condoms and not knowing where and how condoms can be obtained. Even under circumstances where people would like to use condoms, a steady supply is not always available, especially in rural areas.

Provider barriers

Intentionally or not, healthcare providers can strongly influence the availability and acceptability of condoms in their communities. Providers are generally interested in family planning methods that are fast, effective and require little counselling or follow-up. Worldwide, only 2 per cent of couples rely on condoms for family planning, because of the availability of other highly effective methods that are less awkward to use. Providers may even encourage or discourage clients from using certain methods based on their personal opinion of how compliant that client will be, favouring hormonal methods such as Norplant, Depo-Provera or oral contraceptives. The correct use of condoms, in contrast, requires counselling and demonstration, and necessitates a discussion of both family planning and STD prevention. Finally, family planning providers for years have been taught that condoms are relatively ineffective, and this notion probably continues to be conveyed to their clients.

Political barriers

Condom promotion and condom use cannot be successful in any setting without the tacit or preferably vocal support of local and national leaders. The mass-media promotion of condoms through social marketing programmes has been shown not only to increase condom use, but also to improve the visibility and public image of condoms. Where condom advertising is restricted, or is only targeted to married couples, there is little to contradict the negative myths that are often widespread. For example, some of the student-led anti-AIDS clubs in Zambia do not support the promotion of condoms, fearing that they will be an excuse for promiscuity.[14]

Economic barriers

Although many condoms are distributed for free or are sub-sidised by social marketing programmes, the cost of a steady condom supply is still not possible for the very poor. Despite the great success of social marketing, as prices slowly increase the poorest will no longer be able to afford condoms.

Strategies for increasing condom availability and accessibility

- Conduct thorough formative or market research before intro-ducing a variety or brand of condom through the public or private sector.
- Continue to promote mass-media messages and condom social marketing programmes which, in addition to supplying con-doms, make condoms more visible and acceptable.
- Advocate for changes in laws and policies that restrict condom sales to only certain populations.
- Promulgate better understanding of how negotiation/commu-nication skills help women to increase condom use within marriage.
- Pursue research on men's role in condom use. Negotiation skills directed at women alone will not be sufficient for increas-ing condom use within marriage.
- Reconcile inconsistencies in messages on condoms for family planning and disease prevention   condom promotion for family planning influences condom promotion for HIV and vice versa.
- Expand the number of condom outlets   private, public, out-reach, community-based distribution, pharmacies, clinics etc. – while making sure that those outlets reduce the distance that people are required to travel to obtain condoms.[15]
- Emphasize the attributes of condoms that users think are important and base marketing around these attributes, rather than promoting condoms based on safety and efficacy alone.

References

1 Gardner R, Blackburn R, Upadhyay U. *Closing the condom gap*. Population Reports, Series H, No. 9. Baltimore: Johns Hopkins University School of Public Health, Population Information Program, April 1999.
2 Mehryar A. Condoms: awareness, attitudes and use. In: Cleland J, Ferry B, eds.

Sexual behavior and AIDS in the developing world. London: Taylor and Francis, 1995.

3 Bankole A, Singh S. Couples' fertility and contraceptive decision-making in developing countries: hearing the man's voice. *Int Fam Plann Perspect* 1998; **24**(1): 15–24.

4 Agha S. Sexual activity and condom use in Lusaka, Zambia. *Int Fam Plann Perspect* 1998; **24**(1): 32–7.

5 Rwabukwali CB, Schumann DA, McGrath JW *et al*. Culture, sexual behavior and attitudes toward condom use among Baganda women. In Feldman D, ed. *Global AIDS Policy*. Westport, CT: Bergin and Garvey, 1994.

6 Lamptey PR, Coates TJ. Community-Based AIDS Interventions in Africa. In: Essex M *et al*., eds, *AIDS in Africa*. New York: Raven Press, 1994.

7 McGrath JW, Rwabukwali CB, Schumann, DA *et al*. Anthropology and AIDS: The cultural context of sexual risk behavior among urban Baganda women in Kampala, Uganda. *Soc Sci Med* 1993; **36**: 429–39.

8 Murphy JS. *The condom industry in the United States*. McFarland & Co., 1990.

9 Goodkind D, Anh PT. Comment: reasons for rising condom use in Vietnam. *Int Fam Plann Perspect* 1997; **23**(4): 173–8.

10 Cohen B, Trussell J, eds. Preventing and Mitigating AIDS in Sub-Saharan Africa: research and data priorities for the social and behavioral sciences. Washington, DC: National Academy Press, 1996.

11 McNeil ET, Gilmore CE, Finger WR, Lewis JH, Schellstede WP, eds. *The Latex Condom*. North Carolina: Family Health International, 1998.

12 Knodel J, Pramualratana A. Prospecs for increased condom use within marriage in Thailand. *Int Fam Plann Perspect* 1996; **22**: 97–102.

13 Lear, D. Women and AIDS in Africa: A critical review. In: Subedi J, Gallagher EB, eds. *Society, health, and disease: transcultural perspectives*. Englewood-Cliffs: Prentice Hall, 1996, 276–301.

14 Webb D. *HIV and AIDS in Africa*. London: Pluto Press, 1997.

15 Lamptey PR, Price JE. Social Marketing Sexually Transmitted Disease and HIV Prevention: a consumer-centered approach to achieving behavior change. *AIDS* 1997; **12**(Suppl 2), S1–S9.

Further reading

Anderson JE, Cheney R, Clatts M *et al*. HIV risk behavior, street outreach, and condom use in eight high-risk populations. *AIDS Educ Prevent* 1996; **8**(3): 191–204.

Schoepf BG. Culture and AIDS Prevention in Africa. In: Ten Brummelheis H, Herdt G, eds. *Culture and sexual risk: anthropological perspectives on AIDS*. Gordon and Breach, 1995, 29–51.

Steiner M, Piedrahita C, Glover L, Joanis C. Can condom users likely to experience condom failure be identified? *Family Planning Perspectives* 1993; **25**: m220–224 and 226.

Williamson NE, Joanis C. Acceptability of barrier methods for prevention of unwanted pregnancy and infection. In: Mauck CK, Cordero M, Gablenick HL, Speiler JM, Rivera R, eds, Barrier contraceptives: Current Status and Future Prospects, Proceedings of the 4th Contraceptive Research and Development Program International Workship. 1993 March 22–25; Santo Domingo, Dominican Republic. New York: Wiley-Liss, 1993, 53–67.

12 Design and manufacture of male non-latex condoms for prevention of pregnancy and STIs

GASTON FARR

The AIDS pandemic has led to extensive research and development efforts directed to finding alternative materials for condom manufacture. These materials are being evaluated for many reasons. First, an ever increasing number of complaints of allergic reactions to impurities or components in latex material have been reported, most notably among health care workers using latex gloves and to a lesser extent among men and women after using latex condoms.[1-9] Second, latex condoms are weakened and more likely to fail when oil-based lubricants such as baby oils, hand lotions, and petroleum jelly are used.[10] Finally, when latex condoms are stored where it is difficult to prevent high temperatures and exposure to ultraviolet light (i.e. tropical climates), shortened shelf-life and increases in breakage may result if they are not packaged in improved and expensive materials.[11]

In spite of the fact that latex condoms offer protection against pregnancy and sexually transmitted infections (STIs) when used consistently and correctly, many men and women choose to have unprotected intercourse or use another contraceptive method rather than electing to use a condom. Reasons for not using latex condoms are varied, with the most frequently mentioned being[12]:

- lack of sensation or reduced sexual pleasure
- psychological and social factors, including couple communication and assumptions that condoms are for use in extramarital affairs and with sex workers
- lack of availability of condoms, including policies that prohibit condom distribution to youth

- lack of confidence in the reliability of condoms themselves.

While most condom users rarely experience failure, certain behaviours may lead to increased risk of latex condom breakage and/ or slippage. Improper storage, rough handling of condoms, improper donning techniques, lack of natural vaginal lubrication, using excessive added lubrication, use of oil-based lubricants, lengthy or vigorous sex, loss of erection prior to withdrawal, and re-use of condoms all lead to an increased risk of latex condom breakage or slippage.[12] Development of materials that resist breakage and slippage, do not deteriorate when stored under adverse conditions, and are more comfortable and allow greater sensation, may increase condom effectiveness and use.

Until the mid-1990s, consumers using a condom to protect against unwanted pregnancy and/or STIs had only two choices: natural membrane (i.e. lambskin), or latex rubber condoms. Although natural membrane condoms may not be considered very effective in preventing the transmission of STIs, they still offer an option for protection against pregnancy. Latex condoms come in a variety of styles, shapes, colours, and thickness; they may contain spermicide, plain lubricant, or no lubricant. Non-latex condoms offer different design and material characteristics that may have advantages over both natural membrane and latex condoms. Materials used in non-latex condoms are believed to:[12]

- be stronger than latex condoms
- be better able to transmit body heat and improve sexual sensation
- not have the odour often reported for latex condoms
- be more homogeneous allowing for better quality control during manufacture
- not deteriorate under adverse storage conditions
- be less likely to result in allergic reactions, especially among those allergic to latex and/or its component materials
- be more comfortable and easier to use
- be formulated to feel as if they are thinner than they actually are
- be used with a wider variety of lubricants that are more often available to users.

The first non-latex male condom made its appearance on consumer shelves in the United States in 1994, and thereafter in the United Kingdom and Europe. This condom (Avanti, London

International Group), along with others that are currently in development or about to be marketed, will offer additional condom options for couples to meet their contraceptive and sexual health needs, while hopefully leading to more widespread use.

Currently available products and material options

Owing to the proprietary climate that currently characterises product research and development, details about non-latex condom materials and manufacturing processes are limited. What is generally known is that male non-latex condoms are being fabricated using either a dip-mould process or a cut-and-seal process.[12] Non-latex condoms produced using the dipping process generally take on the same appearance of standard male latex condoms and are donned by being unrolled onto the penis. They utilise various ring-type designs for retention on the penis, since currently used synthetic materials do not possess the elastic properties of latex. Condoms made with a cut-and-seal process make use of films extruded from various synthetic materials and can also take on the appearance of standard latex condoms. However, one current design utilises a two-layer flange or collar for retention, a marked departure from the traditional male condom design.

Three different types of materials are currently being used for these condoms: polyester polyurethanes, polyether polyurethanes, and styrene based elastomers. Most result in a condom that is as thin as latex and one that is coated with either a water or silicone based lubricant.

Five non-latex synthetic male condoms have received clearance for marketing in the United States under the Food and Drug Administration's 510(k) substantial equivalence process. Only one, the Avanti polyurethane condom, is available commercially in the United States. Two synthetic condoms under the Trojan brand name (Carter-Wallace, Inc.) and two Tactylon® brand condoms (Sensicon, Inc.) have been cleared but are not available to consumers at the time of this writing. Other non-latex condoms under various stages of development for the US market are the eZ•on® condom from Mayer Laboratories, Inc. and a polyurethane condom from Ortho-McNeil Pharmaceutical of Canada. Avanti and eZ•on® have obtained the CE mark and are now being sold in Europe. Sagami Rubber Industries, Inc.

has marketed a dipped polyurethane condom in Japan under the brand name Sagami Original. Also, a polyethylene condom is being marketed in Colombia under the brand name Unique, with limited distribution in Latin America. Little information is currently available regarding the last two products.

Product development issues

Evaluation and testing of non-latex materials for condom manufacture has represented an exhaustive effort involving considerable time and resources. Development and installation of mass production equipment and intensive quality control systems, along with extensive preclinical and clinical testing for regulatory submissions not previously required for latex condoms, are factors that developers must confront to bring non-latex condoms to market. Grappling with an expansive latex condom market – in 1997 there were over 100 different latex condoms products marketed in the United States alone – manufacturers must also weigh enormous developmental and production costs against an unknown potential market demand in deciding whether to pursue a non-latex condom alternative.

Non-latex condoms also have different physical, stability, and toxicological characteristics than do latex condoms. Standard physical test methods for latex condoms (i.e. ASTM D-3492, CEN600, ISO 4074, etc.) are inappropriate for non-latex condoms.[13] Establishing minimum requirements for air inflation, elongation and tensile strength testing used for latex condoms has also proven to be challenging and problematic. For example, elastomers currently being used for non-latex condoms do not stretch like conventional latex condoms. As a result, many polyurethane condoms break at lower air volume (but higher air pressure) than latex condoms. Added to this is the variety of synthetic materials being used which makes development of a single set of standards a complex and difficult task. International standards for the physical testing of latex condoms have served as references for specifications for testing of non-latex condoms. Work is underway to identify common areas for standards, and the American Society for Testing Materials (ASTM) has established a Task Group on Synthetic Condoms comprised of representatives of condom manufacturers to develop test methods for non-latex condoms. Manufacturers of non-latex condoms are expected to adhere to these standards once they have been developed (see Figures 12.2 and 12.3).

Preclinical and clinical requirements for approval to market non-latex condoms

Prior to 1995, US condom developers used individualised research and development programmes to establish claims of substantial equivalence to meet the general requirements outlined under Title 21 of the US Code of Federal Regulations. To help standardise the evaluation of new condoms, the US Food and Drug Administration's (FDA) Obstetrics–Gynecology Devices Branch issued a draft document, *Testing Guidance for Male Condoms Made from New Material*, in 1995.[18] This document serves as FDA's direction concerning the preclinical and clinical research and documentary procedures needed for marketing clearance.

This guidance document also provides a blueprint for conducting a comprehensive clinical research programme for establishing the functional, safety and contraceptive efficacy parameters for these condoms. It includes recommendations for information needed on: condom sheath and retention mechanism material(s); manufacturing processes; material toxicity; finished product (i.e. description of device and physical testing requirements); quality control and quality assurance; packaging; barrier properties, permeability and shelf-life; as well as clinical data requirements, and study design suggestions.

To obtain regulatory clearance for marketing new non-latex condoms in the United States, the guidance states that:

> . . . the material design, and laboratory performance of the new male condom should be thoroughly studied prior to beginning any clinical studies. Results from the preclinical and clinical studies must demonstrate that the safety and effectiveness of the new condom is substantially equivalent to a legally marketed condom in order to proceed through the premarket notification process.[14]

The FDA guidance document requires that a "slippage and breakage study of sufficient sample size for a statistically valid comparative analysis of the study condom to a legally marketed condom" be completed prior to marketing.[14] The guidance also requires that a contraceptive effectiveness study be conducted comparing the new condom to a marketed latex condom "because there are no validated models to predict the contraceptive effectiveness of a new condom from other clinical performance such as breakage and slippage rates".[14]

Owing to the urgent public health need for alternatives to latex condoms, FDA is allowing flexibility as to when a sponsor conducts the contraceptive effectiveness study. A sponsor may submit an FDA 510(k) application for premarket clearance at the completion of the breakage and slippage study prior to completing the contraceptive effectiveness trial. However, if cleared for marketing, the new condom can only be labelled "*For Latex Sensitive Users Only*", and cannot include statements regarding contraceptive or prophylactic properties.[14] A contraceptive effectiveness trial could then be performed as a post-market study for obtaining unrestricted labelling (i.e. comparable to that of latex condoms claiming that the condom protects against pregnancy and STIs). Because of this labelling restriction, some sponsors may choose to conduct the contraceptive effectiveness study in a premarket setting (i.e. before a 510(k) is cleared for the product). In this case, however, the FDA considers the contraceptive effectiveness study to be a significant risk device investigation that must be conducted under the investigational device exemption (IDE) regulations. Because of the amount of time a contraceptive effectiveness study requires, US developers must weigh the importance of getting to market quickly versus obtaining the less restrictive labelling.

In May 1996, the United Nations Development Program (UNDP), the United Nations Population Fund (UNFPA), the World Health Organization (WHO) and the World Bank Special Programme of Research, Development and Research Training in Human Reproduction, in collaboration with the Rockefeller Foundation and the Wellcome Trust, convened a consultation in Geneva, Switzerland to evaluate international requirements for new condom development. Representatives included condom developers, manufacturers, regulators and researchers.

As an outgrowth of this meeting, WHO issued in 1997 a report titled: *Preclinical and clinical requirements for approval to market non-latex condoms*,[15] with recommendations for the type of information that should be required for regulatory approval of non-latex condoms throughout the world in a timely and cost-effective manner. Some of the recommendations differ from those of the FDA guidance.[14] Meeting participants recommended the following:[15]

1 Contraceptive efficacy trials are not needed to provide assurances that new non-latex condoms are as safe and effective as latex condoms. There was no compelling reason to expect significantly different rates of contraceptive efficacy if breakage and slippage rates of the new condoms gathered in a statistically valid study were equivalent or lower than those of conventional latex condoms. Post-marketing surveillance, however, would be useful to monitor in-use experience, unplanned pregnancies, genital irritation and other adverse events.

2 Labelling similar to that for latex condoms should be allowed for impermeable non-latex condoms when breakage and slippage rates are at least equivalent to those of conventional latex condoms that meet international testing standards (e.g. CEN600, ISO 4074). Additional substantial claims, such as the degree of contraceptive protection, may be allowed if statistically valid data are provided.

3 Package labelling of all condoms should provide a more positive message to consumers, referring more to their ability to protect against pregnancy or STIs, rather than on potential disclaimers and warnings.

4 Protocols for premarket breakage and slippage studies should adopt standardised procedures and definitions of breakage and slippage in order to provide for more cross-study comparison.[15]

The WHO and FDA guidance documents differed principally along the first two recommendations above. The FDA specified a comparative contraceptive efficacy study to provide assurance that the safety and efficacy of a non-latex condom are not inferior to those of a conventional latex condom. Unlike the FDA, the WHO recommended that a comparative breakage and slippage study (i.e. having at least 1 000 uses of the control and 1 000 uses of the test condoms where each couple uses at least 3–5 condoms of each type) is adequate for this purpose.[15] Unlike the FDA, WHO advises that generic labelling similar to that for latex condoms is appropriate if adequate breakage and slippage data are available.

Currently there are no specific regulatory requirements for development and testing of non-latex condoms within the European Economic Area. After 15 June, 1998 all non-latex male condoms have fallen under the regulatory requirements established in the Medical Device Directive (MDD). All medical devices falling under the scope of the Directive must meet certain essential health, safety and administrative requirements based on process controls and safety and effectiveness data provided by manufacturers in their Device Master Files. Until the European Committee for Standardisation (CEN) prescribes a standard for non-latex condoms, condom manufacturers wishing to market non-latex condoms in the United Kingdom and Europe will need to obtain the CE mark to demonstrate compliance with existing medical device requirements.

Published human use studies

Data are emerging on rates of breakage and slippage for male non-latex condoms, mainly for the Avanti polyurethane condom, the first widely marketed polyurethane condom.[16-19]

Prior to marketing of the product, the manufacturer of the Avanti condom commissioned a series of four independent breakage and slippage studies of its product.[16] While the Avanti underwent design changes over the course of these studies, the clinical breakage rates ranged 0.3–2.1 per cent, and the complete slippage rate ranged 1.0–3.5 per cent (Table 12.1). Only one of these studies (Study 1) compared the functional performance of the Avanti condom to that of a marketed latex condom. In this particular study, the clinical breakage rate for the latex comparator was 2.1 per cent, while the complete slippage rate was 1.3 per cent. Due to the small sample size, the difference in breakage rates was not statistically significant.

Five small studies comparing the Avanti condom and a latex control were done between 1991 and 1994 by the Los Angeles Regional Family Planning Council (now the California Family

Table 12.1 Preliminary clinical studies of the Avanti[TM] condom in England (commissioned by London International Group)[a]

Study	Users/ couples	Total uses	Clinical breakage rate	Complete slippage rate	Clinical failure rate
Study 1	188	469	0.9	1.3	2.1
Study 2 – *Condom A*	199	481	1.7	2.4	4.2
Study 2 – *Condom B*	199	472	2.1	1.0	3.2
Study 3	208	548	1.1	1.1	2.2
Study 4	244	670	0.3	3.5	3.9

Source: [a] Adapted from Rosenberg MJ, *et al.*

Health Council, or CFHC) under a grant from the National Institute of Child Health and Human Development (NICHD).[17] Breakage rates ranged from 4.4 to 15 per cent for the Avanti condom and from 0.9 to 2.3 per cent for the latex condom, respectively (Table 12.2). These small studies lacked sufficient power to detect significant differences, however, and a larger, more powerful comparative study was initiated by the CFHC in 1995 and completed in 1997.[18]

A total of 360 couples used 3 of the Avanti polyurethane condoms and 3 latex condoms for sexual intercourse. The clinical breakage rate of the Avanti condom was 7.2 per cent, compared to 1.1 per cent for the latex comparator, while the complete slippage rate was 3.6 and 0.8 per cent, respectively.[18] The breakage and slippage rates for Avanti were significantly greater than for the latex device (Table 12.3, Panel 1).

CFHC also conducted a study of the contraceptive effectiveness, acceptability and safety of the Avanti condom with a standard, commercially available latex condom from 1993 through to 1996.[19] As part of this study, couples completed detailed usage reports for each of the first five acts of vaginal intercourse with the study condoms they were assigned to use. A total of 805 couples were enrolled, with 401 randomised to use the polyurethane condom and 404 the latex condom as their sole means of contraception during the course of the 6-month study.

The clinical breakage rate for the Avanti condom was 4.0 per cent, compared to 0.4 per cent for the latex comparator, while the complete slippage rates were 1.2 and 0.2 per cent, respectively (Table 12.3, Panel 2).[19] The differences in the clinical breakage and complete slippage rates between the Avanti and latex condoms group were statistically significant ($p < 0.001$). While the

Table 12.2   Results of preliminary clinical studies of the Avanti[TM] condom in Los Angeles (NIH)

Study (Date)[a]	Couples	Total uses	Clinical breakage rate[b]
Study 1 (9/91)	24	226	15.0
Study 2 (7/92)	26	243	9.0
Study 3 (9/92)	19	96	5.0
Study 4 (3/93)	20	97	9.0
Study 5 (9/94)	39	114	4.0

Source: [a] *AIDS Alert* 1995; **10**(5): 63. [b] The term "Clinical Breakage Rate" in this table was substituted "Tear Rate".

Table 12.3   Clinical breakage and slippage rates for the Avanti[TM] and latex condoms: California Family Health Council studies, 1995 to 1997

Clinical failure rates	Polyurethane		Latex		Risk Ratio (95% CI)
	N	%	N	%	
Breakage/slippage study[a]					
Total condoms used	1025		1001		
Clinical Breakage	74	7.2	11	1.1	6.6 (3.5–12.3)
Complete Slippage	37	3.6	6	0.8	6.0 (2.6–14.2)
Total Clinical Failure	111	10.8	17	1.7	6.4 (3.9–10.5)
Nested Breakage/Slippage (Contraceptive Effectiveness Study)[b]					
Total condoms used	1804		1882		
Clinical Breakage	72	4.0	8	0.4	9.4 (4.5–19.4)
Complete Slippage	22	1.2	3	0.2	7.7 (2.3–25.2)
Total Clinical Failure	94	5.2	11	0.6	8.9 (4.8–16.6)

Sources: [a] Frezieres RG, et al.[18] [b] California Family Health Council.[19]

results from the nested breakage and slippage component indicated that the Avanti condom failed (broke or slipped off) more frequently during intercourse or withdrawal than did the latex condom; 6-month typical use contraceptive failure rates were not statistically different (Avanti 4.6 ± 2.3 per cent, latex 6.1 ± 2.6 per cent, $p = 0.52$). Avanti condom users did experience a proportionally higher 6-month consistent use pregnancy rate (2.6 ± 2.2 per cent) than did latex condom users (1.0 ± 1.4 per cent), but the difference was not statistically different due to the low numbers of pregnancies among consistent users.[19]

Several studies of the incidence of breakage and slippage of the Tactylon® condom (Sensicon Corporation, USA), a hypoallergenic non-latex polymer condom, have been completed.[20–22] In a study conducted by Trussell et al.[20] among 49 couples who used Tactylon and Trojan-Enz® latex condoms during protected vaginal intercourse, 7 (1.5 per cent) of 478 Tactylon condoms broke or slipped completely off the penis, compared to 2 (0.4 per cent) of 471 Trojan-Enz condoms. However, these differences were not statistically significant given the study size and number of condoms used.[20] In an unpublished study comparing approximately 500 uses of 3 Tactylon designs (standard "latex-like" design, a more elastic, low-modulus design, and a "baggy" design) with 560 uses of a latex condom, the combined clinical breakage rate of the 3 Tactylon condoms was slightly higher than the latex control.[21]

A recently completed breakage and slippage study conducted by the Contraceptive Research and Development Program (CONRAD), in collaboration with Family Health International (FHI), evaluated 3 different Tactylon® condoms and a latex comparator at 2 US sites.[22] The first type was a standard cylindrical condom having a reservoir tip. The second was a "baggy" condom having an open-end diameter similar to traditional condoms, but with a larger diameter below the open end of the condom to allow for more comfort and pleasure. The third Tactylon condom was a shaped condom with low modulus (low resistance to stretching) and high elongation. The latex comparator was a marketed form-fitting version with a reservoir end.

A total of 443 couples provided data for 1220 Standard Tactylon condoms, 1216 Baggy Tactylon condoms, 1228 Low-Modulus Tactylon condoms, and 1230 latex comparator condoms.[22] Overall, 1143 Standard Tactylon condoms, 1148 Baggy Tactylon condoms, 1175 Low-Modulus Tactylon condoms, and 1166 latex comparator condoms were used for vaginal sex. Clinical breakage (i.e. number of condoms breakage during vaginal intercourse or withdrawal) proportions for each condom type were 3.50 per cent Standard Tactylon condoms, 3.57 per cent Baggy Tactylon condoms, and 4.17 per cent Low-Modulus Tactylon condoms, all at the high end of the range expected for latex condoms. The proportion for the latex condom was 0.86 per cent, the low end of the expected range. The breakage rates for the 3 Tactylon condom types were not equivalent to the Standard Latex condom (Table 12.4). Complete slippage (occurring during

Table 12.4   Condom breakage, complete slippage and failure proportions (P) and their standard errors (SE), CONRAD Tactylon evaluation[a]

Event rates	Standard Tactylon®		Baggy Tactylon®		Low-Modulus Tactylon®		Standard Latex	
	P	SE	P	SE	P	SE	P	SE
Clinical breakage[b]	3.50	0.679	3.57	0.724	4.17	0.678	0.86	0.295
Complete slippage[c]	0.70	0.276	1.31	0.376	0.77	0.305	1.11	0.328

Source: [a] Callahan M et al.[22]   [b] Condom breakage during intercourse or penile withdrawal. [c] A condom slipping completely off the penis during intercourse or during penile withdrawal.

intercourse or withdrawal) proportions were 0.70 per cent for the Standard Tactylon condom, 1.31 per cent for the Baggy Tactylon condom, and 0.77 per cent for the Low-Modulus Tactylon condom, compared to 1.11 per cent for the Standard Latex condom. Slippage rates for the 3 Tactylon condoms were statistically equivalent to the Standard Latex condom (Table 12.4).[22] An unpublished pilot study of the eZ•on condom to provide an early assessment of clinical breakage and complete slippage proportions was conducted in 1997 by Family Health International.[23] One hundred couples were randomly assigned to one of two predetermined condom use sequence groups and were to use 4 condoms (2 eZ•on condoms and 2 standard latex condoms) for four acts of vaginal intercourse over a maximum study period of 2 weeks. Condoms and condom use surveys asking a series of questions about each condom usage were mailed to participants once their eligibility was confirmed and informed consent was received.

Overall, 93 couples completed and returned the condom use surveys, resulting in condom use data for 186 eZ•on and 185 latex condoms (Farr G, personal communication, Family Health International, 1998). Of the 391 condoms opened, 6 eZ•on condoms and 5 latex condoms were not used for intercourse due to inability to don the condom (3 eZ•on condoms and all 5 latex condoms) or to breakage during donning (3 eZ•on condoms). No eZ•on condoms broke during intercourse or penile withdrawal, while 1 latex condom (0.6 per cent) broke during intercourse. Five eZ•on condoms (2.8 per cent) slipped off completely during intercourse or withdrawal, while no latex condoms slipped off. A larger comparative breakage and slippage study of the eZ•on condom is currently ongoing in the United States.

While there is epidemiological evidence that consistent, correct use of latex condoms reduces the overall risk of STIs, to date there are no published studies on the effectiveness of polyurethane condoms in the prevention of STIs. However, *in vitro* testing of the viral permeability of nine unspecified brands of latex condoms and two unspecified polyurethane condoms has been published.[24] Overall, 2.6 per cent of the latex condoms (12 of 470) tested in this study allowed some virus penetration, while 5.3 per cent the polyurethane condoms tested (4 of 76) did so. However, this difference was not statistically different.[23]

Future considerations

Introduction of non-latex condoms into the marketplace is recent, and information is slowly emerging about their acceptability, safety, and effectiveness in actual use. Non-latex condoms potentially offer important advantages over latex condoms, principally their controllable physical properties, uniformity, storability, and lack of allergenic reaction. Whether these condoms will become popular alternatives to latex condoms is still difficult to predict.

Several non-latex male condoms are expected to be available soon in various parts of the world. A lengthy and evolving regulatory review process, coupled with an unpredictable marketplace, still makes it difficult to know how many non-latex male condoms will ultimately be available to consumers. This is especially true in the United States where despite the availability of an expedited review process that would allow early marketing under a restrictive label, non-latex condoms now must be subjected to a long and involved research programme to be considered equivalent to currently marketed latex condoms. Stringent regulatory requirements could inhibit further development of these devices, and may even lead to the abandonment of workable alternatives because of excessive developmental costs and a potentially small share of an already extensive latex condom market.

However, the publication of the 1997 WHO document offers a potentially less restrictive alternative for international regulatory review and approval. Whether countries adopt these recommendations is not yet known, but as more information on the performance and safety of these new devices is gathered, there may be greater movement towards streamlining the regulatory review process in the manner recommended by the WHO. Furthermore, many condom manufacturers continue to develop new non-latex male condoms, despite their potentially higher costs and low initial profitability, because of public health considerations. The availability of non-latex male condoms remains an important public health and family planning goal, and new devices will be introduced in the near future.

References

1 Rademaker M, Forsyth A. Allergic reactions to rubber condoms. *Genitourin Med* 1985; **65**: 194–5.
2 FDA Medical Alert. Allergic reaction of latex containing medical devices. MDA 1992; 91–1: 1–2.
3 Bubank ME. Allergic reactions to latex among health-care workers. *Mayo Clinic Proceedings* 1992; **67**: 1075–9.
4 Fuchs T. Latex allergy. *J Allergy Clin Immuno* 1994; **93**: 951–2.
5 Charous B, Hamilton R, Yunginger J. Occupational latex exposure: characteristics of contact and systemic reactions in 47 workers. *J Allergy Clin Immuno* 1994; **94**: 12–18.
6 Arellano R, Bradley J, Sussman G. Prevalence of latex sensitization among hospital physicians occupationally exposed to latex gloves. *Anesthesiology* 1992; 77: 905–8.
7 Berky Z, Luciano J, James W. Latex glove allergy – a survey of the US Army dental corps. *JAMA* 1992; **268**: 2695–7.
8 Lewis HR. "Sex allergy" may stem from latex condoms. *Med Aspects Hum Sexual* 1991: 11.
9 Stehlin D. Latex allergies: when rubber rubs the wrong way. FDA Consumer 1992: 16–21.
10 Hatcher RA, *et al*. *Contraceptive Technology: Sixteenth Revised Edition*. New York: Irvington Publishers, Inc., 1994: 156–9.
11 Free MJ, Hutchings J, Lubis F, Natakusumah R. An assessment of burst strength distribution data for monitoring quality of condom stocks in developing countries. *Contraception* 1986; **33**: 285–99.
12 McNeill ET, *et al*. eds. *The latex condom: recent advances, future directions*. Research Triangle Park, NC: Family Health International, 1998.
13 Farr G. Clinical research in the development and testing on non-latex condoms: Family Health International's experience from 1987–96. Presented at the Consultation on Pre-Clinical and Clinical Requirements for Non-Latex Male Condoms, World Health Organization, Geneva, Switzerland, May 13–15, 1996.
14 Center for Devices and Radiological Health, Office of Device Evaluation, Division of Reproductive, Abdominal, Ear, Nose and Throat and Radiological Devices, Obstetrics-Gynecology Branch, Food and Drug Administration (FDA). Testing guidance for male condoms made from new material. Washington, DC: FDA, 1995.
15 World Health Organization. Preclinical and clinical requirements for approval to market non-latex condoms: report and recommendations of a WHO Consultation on Preclinical and Clinical Requirements for Non-Latex Male Condoms, Geneva, 13–15 May 1996. Geneva: WHO, 1997.
16 Rosenberg MJ, *et al*. The male polyurethane condom: review of current knowledge. Contraception, 1996;53(3): 141–6.
17 Anonymous. Studies found plastic condom unsafe, yet FDA cleared it for market. *AIDS Alert*, 1995; **10**(5): 61–4.
18 Frezieres RG, Walsh TL, Nelson AL, Clark VA, Coulson AH. Breakage and acceptability of a polyurethane condom: a randomized, controlled study. *Fam Plann Perspect* 1998; **30**(2): 73–8.
19 California Family Health Council. Final Report: Study of the efficacy, acceptability and safety of a non-latex (polyurethane) condom [N01-HD-1-3109]. NICHHD, 1997.
20 Trussell J, Warner DL, Hatcher R. Condom performance during vaginal intercourse: comparison of Trojan-Enz® and Tactylon™ condoms. *Contraception*, 1992; **45**(1): 11–19.

21 Steiner M, Joanis C, Taylor D, *et al.* Final report – functionality and acceptability of three lubricated Tactylon condoms and a standard latex condom.
   Durham, NC: Family Health International, 1993 (unpublished).
22 Callahan M, Mauck C, Taylor D, Wheeless AJ, Frezieres R, Walsh T, Martens
   M, Bellis J. Comparative evaluation of three Tactylon® condoms and a latex
   condom during vaginal intercourse: breakage and slippage. 1999; Recently
   submitted to *AM J Public Health*.
23 Lytle CD, Rouston LB, Seaborn GB, et al. An in-vitro evaluation of condoms
   as barriers to a small virus. *Sexual Transmit Dis*, 1997; **24**(3): 161–4.

13 The female condom

ANNE M YOUNG

Until fairly recently, the latex male condom was the only device widely available which served as both a method of contraception as well as a means to prevent the spread of STIs and HIV. However, in the mid-1980s, the concept of a female condom moved to the design and testing phases. While versions of female condoms had existed as far back as the 1920s, the modern device was invented by Lasse Hessel, a Danish physician, over 10 years ago. The Female Health Company, which is currently the only commercial manufacturer of the female condom, began its development for approval by the US Food and Drug Administration (FDA) in 1987 and obtained the approval for marketing and distribution in May, 1993. The female condom was first launched in Switzerland in 1992, and today the female condom is available in 30 countries in Europe, Africa, Latin America, Asia, the United States and Canada. Current trade names include: Reality®, Femidom® and Femy®; it is marketed under the name of *Care* in several African countries.

The female condom is a strong, soft, transparent sheath made of polyurethane. It is 17 cm long (about the same length as the male condom), 0.042–0.053 mm thick, and 7.8 cm at its widest diameter. The sheath has a flexible ring at either end. The smaller, yet thicker ring at the closed end is used for insertion. It is pre-lubricated with an inert, non-spermicidal, silicone-based fluid called dimethicone lubricant. This lubricant eases the insertion process as well as allowing for a more comfortable movement of the penis. Extra lubrication may be supplied with female condoms sold through the private sector, mainly in the

United States, Canada, and Western Europe. Although the extra lubricant provided is water-based, the integrity of the female condom is not affected by oil-based lubricants such as petroleum jelly or mineral oil. This is important because water-based lubricants are difficult to find in many settings.

The device is inserted much in the way a diaphragm would be introduced into a woman's vagina. The closed end of the female condom covers the cervix and is anchored behind the pubic bone. This ring itself is removable, however removal is not recommended because this could result in the device no longer being anchored in the vagina. The larger and thinner outer ring remains outside the vagina, and anchors the condom so that the sheath covers the labia as well as the base of the penis during intercourse. Thus, while the female condom is in place, it acts as both a protective coating to the vagina as well as a form of partial protection for the external genitalia (see Figure 13.1).

To avoid the penis entering the vagina outside the female condom, it is recommended that one of the partners hold the outer ring of the device in place on the external genitalia. After intercourse, the female condom is removed by twisting the outer ring and pulling it out. By twisting it, semen is trapped in the pouch. As with the male condom, the female condom should be disposed of in a suitable rubbish container, not flushed down a toilet.

Use of the female condom in practice

The female condom was designed to be used during vaginal intercourse as a method of contraception and disease prevention. Now that the female condom has been available for several years, some interesting findings about how it is actually used have emerged. For example, the female condom can also be used by women with vaginal dryness to increase lubrication and reduce painful intercourse (Riley and Riley 1995, unpublished). Other issues emerging are that:

Female condoms are often reused

Each female condom is currently labelled for single use only. However, re-use of the method has been reported in several studies, particularly in the developing world.[1] This is not surprising given that the female condom, even when sold at a subsidised

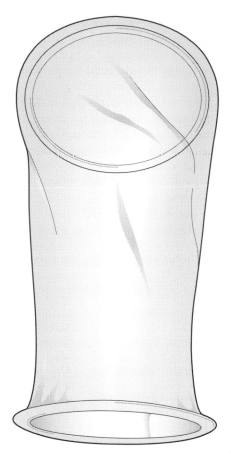

Figure 13.1   The female condom.

price to consumers, is always more expensive than the male condom. Research on the feasibility and safety of re-using the female condom is discussed below.

Female condoms are used in conjunction with male condoms

The practice of using the two condoms concurrently is generally discouraged because the friction generated from inadequate lubrication may cause the male condom to slip off the penis and/or the outer ring of the female condom to be pushed inside the vagina.[2]

Female condoms are used for anal intercourse

The female condom was developed for vaginal intercourse. However, anecdotal evidence and reports by gay men's groups indicate that the female condom is currently being used for anal intercourse among men. The inner ring is usually removed and the condom donned like a male condom. Use of the femal condom for anal intercourse among gay/bisexual men has been confirmed by two unpublished studies (Gross *et al.* 1998, Gibson *et al.* 1999). To date, the use of the female condom for anal intercourse among heterosexual couples has not been explored in the literature.

Physical integrity and safety

The polyurethane used in the manufacture of the female condom is not affected by changes in temperature and humidity, so no special storage conditions are required.[3] The male latex condom, by contrast, can be damaged by heat, light, and humidity.[4] The female condom has been shown to resist deterioration under extreme storage conditions of high temperature and high humidity. The expiration date of the female condom is 60 months (5 years) from the date of manufacture.

Polyurethane is 40 per cent stronger than latex and is less likely to break than latex. Therefore, exposure to semen during use should be minimal or zero if the female condom is used correctly. In studies sponsored by the Female Health Company (formerly Wisconsin Pharmacal) post-coital leak tests showed statistically significant lower rates of leakage among female condom vs. male condoms (0.6 vs. 3.5 per cent respectively).[5,6] With regard to dislodgement of the female condom, these studies found that vaginal exposure to semen occurred among 2.7 per cent of users as compared to a rate of 8.1 per cent for users of the male condom.

Safety

The female condom has been tested for dermal sensitisation and irritation, vaginal irritation, cytotoxicity, and mutagenicity. All studies have shown the female condom to be safe. In a study of vaginal trauma,[7] upon macroscopic and colposcopic examination, scientists found no evidence of trauma associated with use of the female condom, nor were there changes in the vaginal flora. Forsythe (1992) studied the use of the female condom among

120 people with sensitive skin; none of the participants had an irritation or allergic reaction to the device or its lubricant.

As mentioned above, the female condom was designed and labelled for single use only. However, due to the strong demand to reduce the price of the product to consumers, several studies are underway to evaluate the safety of re-using the method. Family Health International (FHI), a US-based research organisation, has been conducting research to determine the physical integrity of the female condom after repeated washings and use. Results of these studies are due to be published in early 2000. Other research sponsored by FHI in Zambia and Bolivia will attempt to ascertain information of the re-use, storage and cleaning patterns currently employed by female condom users.

Some work has already been completed in this area. A study in South Africa suggests that washing, drying, and relubricating the female condom, up to 10 times under a variety of different washing regimes does not significantly alter the device's structural integrity (McIntyre *et al.* 1998, unpublished). In the area of microbial retention of STIs, one study conducted thus far has shown that less than 1 per cent of pathogens were found on female condoms that were artificially inoculated with *Escherishia coli*, *Lactobacillus*, *Gardnerella vaginalis*, *Candida*, *Staphylococcus aureus*, diphtheroids, *Enterococcus*, and Group B *Streptococcus*, and then patted dry after being rinsed with tap water.[8] Even though the findings thus far are promising, the process for obtaining FDA approval for re-use of the device could take several years.

Efficacy of the female condom as a contraceptive

The female condom is intended for contraception and STD prevention. To date, three studies on the contraceptive effectiveness of the female condom have been published. Generally, the efficacy rates discussed in the literature distinguish between perfect use (method used correctly for every act of intercourse) and normal use (where the method is sometimes used incorrectly or not at all). One major study conducted by Farr *et al.*[9] included women from the United States and Latin America. Among the women in the United States a 6-month accidental pregnancy rate was found to be 12.4 per cent with normal use while 2.6 per cent with perfect use. Among the women from Latin America, the overall 6-month accidental pregnancy rate was 22 per cent, with a rate of 9.5 per cent among perfect users. Therefore, the overall rate of pregnancy among women who used the method correctly for every act of intercourse was 4.3 per 100 women over a 6-month period. The limitations of the study design are noted elsewhere.[10]

Another effectiveness study on the female condom was conducted by Bounds et al.[11] in Great Britain. The accidental pregnancy rate (life table) at 12 months was calculated at 15 per cent. The authors concluded that, despite the limitations of the small study, the overall use-effectiveness observed was well within the wide range of that reported for the male condom.

Recent research in Japan by Trussell[12] found that the probability of becoming pregnant within 6 months using the female condom was 3.2 per cent during typical use and 0.8 per cent during correct and consistent use of the female condom. The author noted, however, that the coital frequency among study participants was 59 per cent lower than in the US/Latin American trial, which could account for the lower risk of pregnancy incurred.

The general conclusion is that the female condom provides protection against pregnancy at least as good, if not better, than other barrier methods, including male condoms, the diaphragm, and spermicides.

STI protection

Studies *in vitro* confirm that the female condom can provide an effective barrier to organisms smaller than those known to cause STIs. Independent studies[13,14] as well as those performed by the Female Health Company (performed by the Female Health Company and the British manufacturer Chartex), demonstrate that the female condom provides an effective barrier to gases, liquids and micro-organisms including cytomegalovirus, herpes virus, hepatitis B virus, and HIV. There findings were confirmed by a more recent study by Lytle et al.[15] who concluded that polyurethane condoms provide a substantial barrier to viral transmission. Trussell et al.[16] estimate that perfect use of the female condom may reduce the annual risk of acquiring HIV by more than 90 per cent among women who have intercourse twice weekly with an infected male.

Soper et al.[17] studied the female condom's protective effect against re-infection among a group of 104 women who had been diagnosed with vaginal trichomoniasis and found that among those women who used the method with every act of intercourse, none experienced a re-occurrence of vaginal trichomoniasis.

A study by the United Nations Programme on AIDS (UNAIDS) in Thailand showed that use of the female condom can lead to a reduction in STIs.[18] Some groups of commercial sex workers were given male condoms only; others were given both male and female condoms. Among those supplied with both female and male condoms, the number of unprotected sex acts was 25 per cent lower than among those only receiving male condoms. In addition, there was also a 34 per cent reduction in the mean incidence rate of STIs among those with access to both types of condoms. Unpublished research conducted in Philadelphia found that female condoms were equally as effective as male condoms at preventing STIs. After study participants were supplied either male or female condoms, follow-up showed 18 and 19 per cent re-infection rates respectively over a 6-month period (French et al. 1998, unpublished). However, the results were contradicted in another study in Zimbabwe (Mason et al. 1996, unpublished) where commercial sex workers were assigned randomly to receive supplies and education on female and male condoms (group A) or male condoms only (group B). The authors found little difference between the two groups in terms of STI acquisition (37 per cent in group A and 39 per cent in group B); however, women in group A were likely to be free of STIs for longer than those in group B. The outcome can likely be explained by the fact that women in both groups used the condom inconsistently due to difficulty negotiating its use with partners.

The conclusion that can be drawn from the limited research to date is that the female condom can provide an effective physical barrier to the passage of STIs, including the HIV virus. In addition, when female condoms are offered as an alternative or additional method to male condoms, choice is enhanced and the number of protected sexual acts increases, hence reducing the rate of disease transmission. However, as with any barrier method, the effectiveness in preventing the spread of disease is dependent on the correct and consistent use of the method.

Acceptability of the female condom

In 1997, the WHO and UNAIDS conducted a comprehensive review of the existing literature on the female condom.[19] This included efficacy and acceptability research carried out to date.

This review was intended to help the agencies make strategic decisions about the wide scale, global introduction of the female condom. In early 1998, another comprehensive literature review was compiled by Cecil et al.[20]

The overall finding of the various studies on acceptability of the female condom is that it is highly acceptable in many contexts among a variety of different ethnic and social groups.[21-25] (Klein et al. 1998; Klackmann et al. 1998; Sankaran et al. 1998; Surrat et al. 1998, unpublished).

However, the research undertaken thus far suffers from several weaknesses. Many studies are presented at international conferences but have not been published in peer review journals and are thus seen as less credible. Cecil et al.[26] provide a comprehensive critique of the study limitations. Most studies have involved small sample sizes, have suffered from high attrition rates, and have focused only on those who were willing to use the method. Little research on attitudes has been conducted among those who are *unwilling* to use the method. In addition, most studies have employed cross-sectional designs; less than half a dozen recent studies have followed up women or couples for 6 months or more, to measure change in attitudes and behaviours in relation to the female condom in the long term. Little information has emerged as to the specific factors associated with use or non-use of the method, or the demographic and psychosocial factors that can predict use.

What has emerged so far is that positive and negative aspects of the female condom tend to vary by cultural context. What may be considered a major advantage of the method in one culture serves as a deterrent to its use in another. Leeper and Stein[27] point to the example of lubrication; in settings where extra lubricant is appreciated, the female condom with its high degree of lubrication may be quite acceptable. However, the method may be rejected in cultures where dry sex is desirable. Often the acceptability of the method can be correlated with the acceptability of contraception (in particular barrier methods) and disease prevention in general. The positive and negative aspects of the method found from acceptability studies was summarised in *The female condom: a review*[28] (See Table 13.1).

Table 13.1   Positive and negative aspects of using the female condom

Positive	Negative
Increases sexual stimulation; feels warm	Reduces sexual pleasure
Internal ring stimulates with rubbing and orgasm is reached more quickly	The outer part of the condom covers the clitoris and inhibits orgasm
Women gain power and control	Men are absolved of responsibility
Provides opportunity for communication about sex, pregnancy, STIs/HIV	Women are unable to discuss it with partners (as with the male condom), or men will refuse to use it
Insertion/use becomes easier over time and with experience	Difficult to insert; causes frustration and quick abandonment of method
Lubrication reduces pain during intercourse	Too much lubrication; makes insertion difficult; not appropriate in contexts where dry sex is valued
Very clean feeling after using method because ejaculate remains in the condom, which can be removed after intercourse	Is messy
Does not interrupt erotic play and no risk of partner losing his erection because it can be inserted ahead of time. Can be eroticised	Interrupts lovemaking; not spontaneous; requires forethought/ planning
Non-constricting	Internal ring painful for both partners
Odourless and tasteless	Noisy
Less likely to slip or break compared to latex male condom; stronger than male condom	Expensive
Can use multiple forms of lubrication	May not be appropriate for all sexual positions; appears to work best in the "missionary position"
Soft, non-drying texture	Too large; aesthetically unpleasant; looks like a plastic bag
Makes women feel safe, secure	Penis can enter vagina outside the female condom or push the whole condom inside vagina
Reduces need to hurry to have the partner withdraw after intercourse out of fear of it slipping off while inside the vagina thus prolonging intimacy	Arouses suspicion of infidelity; raises issues of trust; may lead to violent reaction from male partner

Comparison of female and male condoms

Both the male and female condom offer good protection against pregnancy and STIs when used properly. The female condom has been used only in the past few years and studies are still quite limited (as dicussed above). However, the female condom can potentially have some advantages over the male condom. For example, the polyurethane used in the female condom is stronger than latex. Breakage rarely occurs and this affords couples confidence in the product. The female condom can be used with multiple forms of lubrication. Whereas latex deteriorates with the use of oil-based lubricants such as cooking oil or petroleum jelly, the female condom will not deteriorate with the use of these lubricants.

In addition, the female condom does not cause allergic reactions. While up to 8 per cent of people are allergic to the latex used to manufacture the male condom,[29] allergic reactions to polyurethane have not been reported anywhere in the literature. Theoretically, the female condom should offer greater protection from pathogens because it covers external as well as internal genitalia. However, this has not yet been scientifically proven.

Unlike the male condom, the female condom can be inserted several minutes to several hours before intercourse and does not require an erect penis for placement. In addition, it does not have to be removed immediately after ejaculation when the penis becomes flaccid. This allows the couple to stay together longer after the male orgasm has been achieved which could enhance intimacy.

The female condom can be used without knowledge or consent of the male partner. Because of economic, social and gender inequalities, women are often not in a position to get their partners to use male condoms.[30,31] Although ideally used with the co-operation of the male partner, the female condom has been noted as highly advantageous in situations where the negotiation of the male condom is impossible. In some research, especially among commercial sex workers, clients are not even aware that the female condom is in place.

Like the male condom, the female condom can be supplied "over the counter" or through community-based distribution. The device does not require fitting or refitting unlike the diaphragm, and does not require a visit to a health professsional. However, for first time users, it helps to have advice about insertion and use from another user or a trained provider.

Currently the female condom is more expensive that the male condom in all settings. In developing countries where the price has put the female condom closer to the cost of other methods, it has been very popular (see discussion below). However, in the United States, for example, the high cost of the method in comparison with the male condom could be a barrier for couples, especially adolescents.[32]

The female condom: present and future

The initial demand for female condoms has been strong; in some instances, the acceptance of the female condom has been quite unexpected. An example from Zimbabwe is illustrative. There, men generally still control many aspects of social and sexual life. Nevertheless, in 1996, more than 30 000 women petitioned the country's government to make the method available on a wide scale. The number sold in the first three months of introduction was four times that expected.[33] Zimbabwe has the highest rate of HIV infection in the world; so strong is the need for women and men to protect themselves that social and cultural barriers to condom use have been eroded.

Demand for the female condom is obviously affected by cost. There is currently a three-tiered pricing structure for the female condom. The first is through the private sector where the female condom is available for purchase between US$2–3. The female condom is currently available through the private sectors in Antigua, Taiwan, Republic of Korea, South Africa, Thailand, the United States, Canada, Holland, Spain, Switzerland, and the United Kingdom.

In Europe and the United States, interest in the method is on the rise. Market research in Great Britain indicates that 1 per cent of women aged 18–45 use the female condom as their main method of contraception. This is comparable to the use of the diaphragm which has been available for decades. The Female Health Company reports that it has sold over eight million female condoms in the United States since it was first marketed in 1994. The majority of outlets are family planning establishments but there is now growing interest among HIV/AIDS prevention programmes. However, one study in the United States, conducted with 413 STD clinic clients, indicates that while three-quarters of participants had heard of the method, less than 6 per cent knew of any one who had used it and only 2.7 per cent had tried it themselves.[34] Hence the market potential in the United States is still being discovered.

In 1996, the United Nations Programme on AIDS (UNAIDS) sent an initial survey to all developing countries to assess the demand for the female condom at a reduced price. Over 50 countries responded and expressed an expected demand for 13 million condoms in 1998, if the method were available at a reasonable price. The unit cost for developing countries was reduced from US$2 to $0.62 through UNAIDS' negotiation with the Female Health Company. This has made the female condom a realistic option for developing countries.

Today, the female condom is available at subsidised prices to social marketing organisations in a number of developing countries including Bolivia, Kenya, Zambia, and Zimbabwe. Through this system, the method is available through retail outlets and community-based distributors at a greatly reduced price to the consumer (two condoms for less than $0.25 in Zambia and Zimbabwe, for example).

In addition, the female condom is being purchased by Ministries of Health and supplied free of charge in public clinics. Large shipments of the female condom have been made to Brazil, Kenya, South Africa, Tanzania, Uganda, Venezuela, Zambia, and Zimbabwe. Other countries who are still studying acceptability and introduction strategies have made smaller orders; these include Cameroon, Côte d'Ivoire, Costa Rica, Eritrea, Ghana, Indonesia, and Papua New Guinea.

It is important to note that many countries have reordered the female condom after an initial shipment in 1997. This indicates that there is indeed high demand for the method and that Ministries of Health are willing to invest their overstretched resources in this product.

Because of the study design limitations discussed above, and the relatively short time since the method was introduced globally, it is hard to predict the long-term role of the female condom in expanding contraceptive choice and disease prevention options. Only one study to date has followed couples one year after enrolment. This was conducted in Zambia and was able to follow two-thirds of the couples. The research found that couples used the female condom for just less than 25 per cent of coital acts.[35] The proportion of couples using the female condom decreased over time while the proportion of coital acts protected remained stable. Continuity of use was greater where the risk of acquiring STIs/HIV was perceived to be greater (for example, where only one partner was HIV positive). Hence its use has become more concentrated among fewer couples; it has filled a niche and has resulted in an increase in the proportion of coital acts protected.

Other studies in the United States, United Kingdom, Hong Kong and Kenya have shown that use can be sustained over an extended period. The range of continued use is between 31 and 56 per cent.[36] However, one study (Padian et al. 1998, unpublished) in northern California showed a decreased interest in the female condom over time.

It appears that the novelty phase of the female condom is ending and a phase of serious introduction into a limited market has begun. This market is extremely important because right now the female condom is the only woman-initiated method available for women and men to protect themselves against STIs, including HIV, as well as unwanted pregnancies. Research from several settings has shown that adding the female condom to the arsenal of contraceptive and disease prevention options increases the percentage of protected sexual acts.

Also research shows it has an empowering effect on women in their relationships. The female condom, if introduced in the proper way, can provide a tool in helping women gain more control of their sexual lives and improve relations with their partners. It had been noted that by casting the method as one *initiated* rather than *controlled* by women, it may be less threatening to men and enjoy broader success.[37] This has been the strategy of the social marketing campaign in Zimbabwe; the method has been called the *Care Contraceptive Sheath* to reduce the stigma associated with the word "condom". The product is positioned as a contraceptive method and the slogan reads "*Care* – for women and men who care." Findings from a comprehensive study in Brazil and Kenya reinforce the importance of male acceptance of the method as critical to its success.[38] Communication skills with men were found to be the critical factor for successful female condom use among women participating in qualitative research in four countries.[39] Providing adequate counselling to both men and women on the positive and negative attributes of the device can enhance use.[40] The combination of approaches which have thus far proven effective in introducing the female condom should ideally translate into longer, sustained use of the method and an increase in its popularity.

The latent demand for a female-initiated method of contraception and disease prevention among women worldwide has been uncovered. Supply of this demand had been met and augmented through the concerted efforts of the Female Health Company and UNAIDS. Now other companies are tapping into this demand and other female condoms are being studied and tested. These include a Bikini condom which is worn like a panty, and the "Janesway", which is attached to a female panty in a way that looks like lingerie. This has been developed by the HHH Development Company. In addition, Reddy Medtech Company is field testing a less expensive female condom that employs a sponge in the pouch to keep it in place.[41-43] At the moment, these new models are not available to consumers.

Acknowledgements

I would like to acknowledge the assistance of Jane Cottingham, Technical Officer, Special Programme of Research, Development and Research Training, WHO and Mary Ann Leeper, President of the Female Health Company of Chicago Illinois, who commented on drafts of this chapter. Also the UNDP/UNFPA/WHO/ World Bank Special Programme of Research, Development and Research Training in Human Reproduction for supporting the production of the manuscript *The female condom: a review*, 1997 which served as the background for this report.

Unpublished references

Forsythe A. 1992. Evaluation of the polyurethane female condom (Femidom®) in rubber sensitive individuals and in patients with other skin diseases. Unpublished work presented at the American Society of Dermatology Congress (available from the Female Health Company).

French P, Latka M, Gollub EL, Rogers C, Odonnell J, Stein Z. Female condoms as effective as male condoms in preventing sexually transmitted diseases. Presented at the World AIDS Conference, Geneva, Switzerland, June 1998.

Gross M, Buchbinder SP, Holte S, Celum C, Koblin BA. Use of Reality® condoms for anal sex by HIV-seronegative US gay/bisexual men at increased risk for HIV infection. Presented at the World AIDS Conference, Geneva, Switzerland, June 1998.

Kalckmann S, Rea MF, Villela WV, Vieira EM, Fernandes ME, Andrah EM. Female condom: Exploratory study in Sao Paulo, Brazil. Presented at the World AIDS Conference, Geneva, Switzerland, June 1998.

Klein H, Welka DA, Crosby HL, Eber MR, Hoffman JA. Women substance abusers' concerns about and experiences with the female condom. Presented at the World AIDS Conference, Geneva, Switzerland, June 1998.

Mason P, Ray S, Ndowa F, *et al.* Sexually transmitted diseases and HIV in commercial sex workers supplied with female and/or male condom. Presented at the World AIDS Conference, Vancouver, Canada, July 1996.

McIntyre J, Pettifor A, Rees VH. Female condom re-use: assessing structural integrity after multiple wash, dry and re-lubrication cycles. Presented at the World AIDS Conference, Geneva, Switzerland, June 1998.

Padian N, Quan J, Gould H, Glass S. Choice of the female-controlled method of barrier contraceptives among young women and their male partners in northern California diminishes over time. Presented at the World AIDS Conference, Geneva, Switzerland, June 1998.

Riley A, Riley E. Femidom for superficial dyspareunia. Unpublished report, 1995. (Available from the Female Health Company.)

Sankaran S, Shailaja P, Lalitha S, Kavitha C, Joson M. Acceptability of female condom (FC) as a protective device: a pilot study in India. Presented at the World AIDS Conference, Geneva, Switzerland, June 1998.

Surratt H, Inciardi J, Telles P, McBridge D, Pok B. Acceptability of the female condom among women drug users in Brazil. Presented at the World AIDS Conference, Geneva, Switzerland, June 1998.

Gibson S, McFarland W, Wohlfeiler D, Scheer K, Katz MH. Experiences of 100 men who have sex with men using the Reality condom for anal sex. *AIDS Education and Prevention* 1999. Feb; **11**(1): 65–71.

References

1 UNDP/UNFPA/WHO/World Bank Special Programme of Research, Development and Research Training in Human Reproduction. *The female condom: a review.* Geneva: World Health Organization, 1997.
2 McCabe E, Golub S, Lee AC. Making the female condom a "reality" for adolescents. *J Pediatr Adolesc Gynecol* 1997; **10**: 115–23.
3 UNAIDS. *The female condom and AIDS: UNAIDS point of view,* April 1998.
4 Liskin L, Wharton C, Blackburn R. Condoms – now more than ever. *Popul Rep* 1990; **H**: 1–35.
5 Leeper MA, Conrady M. Preliminary evaluation of REALITY, a condom for women to wear. *Adv Contracept* 1989; **5**: 229–35.
6 Leeper MA. Letters to the Editor: preliminary evaluation of Reality™, a condom for women. *AIDS Care* 1990; **2**: 287–90.
7 Soper DE, Brockwell NJ, Dalton HP. Evaluation of the effects of the female condom on the female lower genital tract. *Contraception* 1991; **44**: 21–9.
8 AIDSCAP. Women's Initiative. Female condom: from research to the marketplace. Chicago: Family Health International, 1997.
9 Farr G, Gabelnick H, Sturgen K, Dorflinger L. Contraceptive efficacy and acceptability of the female condom. *Am J Public Health* 1994; **84**: 1960–4.
10 UNDP/UNFPA/WHO/World Bank Special Programme of Research, Development and Research Training in Human Reproduction. *The female condom: a review.* Geneva: World Health Organization, 1997.
11 Bounds W, Guillebaud J, Newman GB. Female condom (Femidom™). A clinical study of the use-effectiveness and patient acceptability. *Br J Fam Plann* 1992; **18**: 36–41.

12 Trussell J. Contraceptive efficacy of the Reality® female condom. *Contraception* 1998, **55**: 147–8.

13 Drew WL, Blair M, Miner RC, Conant M. Evaluation of the virus permeability of a new condom for women. *Sex Transmit Dis* 1990; **17**: 110–12.

14 Voeller B, Coulter SL, Mayhan KG. Letters to the Editor: gas, dye and viral transport through polyurethane condoms. *JAMA* 1991; **26**: 2986–7.

15 Lytle CD, Routson LB, Seaborn GB, Dixon LG, Bushar HF, Cyr WH. An *in vitro* evaluation of condoms as barriers to a small virus. *Sex Transmit Dis* 1997; **24**: 161–4.

16 Trussell J, Sturgen K, Strickler J, Dominik R. Comparative contraceptive efficacy of the female condom and other barrier methods. *Fam Plann Perspect* 1994; **24**: 66–72.

17 Soper DE, Shoupe D, Shangold GA, *et al.* Prevention of vaginal trichomoniasis by compliant use of the female condom. *Sex Transmit Dis* 1993; **20**: 137–9.

18 Fontanet AL, Saba J, Chandeying V *et al.* Increased protection against sexually transmitted diseases by giving commercial sex workers in Thailand the choice of using the male or female condom: a randomized controlled trial (in press).

19 UNDP/UNFPA/WHO/ World Bank Special Programme of Research, Development and Research Training in Human Reproduction. *The female condom: a review.* Geneva: World Health Organization, 1997.

20 Cecil H, Perry MJ, Seal DW, Pinkerton SD. The female condom: what we have learned thus far. *AIDS Behav* 1998; **2**: 241–56.

21 UNDP/UNFPA/WHO/World Bank Special Programme of Research, Development and Research Training in Human Reproduction. *The female condom: a review.* Geneva: World Health Organization, 1997.

22 Sly DF, Quadagno D, Harrison DF, Eberstein IW, Riehman K, Bailey M. Factors associated with use of the female condom. *Fam Plann Perspect* 1997; **29**: 181–4.

23 Deniaud F. Dynamiques d'acceptabilité du preservatif feminin chez des prostituèes et des jeunes femmes a Abidjan Côte d'Ivoire. *Contracept Fertil Sexual* 1997; **25**: 921–32.

24 Madrigal J, Schifter J, Feldblum PJ. Female condom acceptability among sex workers in Costa Rica. *AIDS Educ Prevent* 1998; **10**: 105–13.

25 Sinpisut P, Chandeying V, Skov S, Uahgowitchai C. Perceptions and acceptability of the female condom [Femidom®] amongst commercial sex workers in the Songkla province, Thailand. *Int J STD AIDS* 1998; **9**: 168–72.

26 Cecil H, Perry MJ, Seal DW, Pinkerton SD. The female condom: what we have learned thus far. *AIDS Behav* 1998; **2**: 241–56.

27 Leeper MA, Stein Z. The female condom: cause and effect of protection. Published Proceedings of the June 1998 World AIDS Conference, Geneva, Switzerland 1998.

28 UNDP/UNFPA/WHO/World Bank Special Programme of Research, Development and Research Training in Human Reproduction. *The female condom: a review.* Geneva: World Health Organization, 1997.

29 UNAIDS. *The female condom and AIDS: UNAIDS point of view,* April 1998.

30 Gollub EL, Stein ZA. Commentary: the new female condom – item 1 on a women's AIDS prevention agenda. *Am J Public Health* 1993; **83**: 498–500.

31 Heise L, Elias C. Transforming AIDS prevention to meet women's needs: a focus on developing countries. *Soc Sci Med* 1995; **40**: 931–43.

32 McCabe E, Golub S, Lee AC. Making the female condom a "reality" for adolescents. *J Pediatr Adolesc Gynecol* 1997; **10**: 115–23.

33 Winter J. Female condom sales beat forecast by 10 times. *AIDS Analysis Africa* 1997; **7**: 9.

34 McGill W, Miller K, Bolan G, *et al.* Letter to the Editor: Awareness of and experience with the female condom among patients attending STD clinics. *Sex Transmit Dis* 1998; **25**: 222–3.

35 Musaba E, Morrison CS, Sunkutu MR, Wong EL. Long-term use of the female condom among couples at high-risk of Human Immunodeficiency Virus infection in Zambia. *Sex Transmit Dis* 1998; **25**: 260–4.

36 Leeper MA and Stein Z. The female condom: cause and effect of protection. Published Proceedings of the June 1998 World AIDS Conference, Geneva, Switzerland 1998.

37 AIDSCAP. Women's Initiative. Female condom: from research to the marketplace. Chicago: Family Health International, 1997.

38 Ankrah EM, Attika SA. Adopting the female condom in Kenya and Brazil: perspectives of women and men, a synthesis. 1997; AIDSCAP, Family Health International.

39 Aggleton P, Rivers K, Scott S. Multi-site studies of gender relations, sexual negotiation, and the female condom in developing countries: a comparative analysis of findings. In press.

40 Musaba E, Morrison CS, Sunkutu MR, Wong EL. Long-term use of the female condom among couples at high-risk of Human Immunodeficiency Virus infection in Zambia. *Sex Transmit Dis* 1998; **25**: 260–4.

41 Anonymous. Developing new diaphragms, condoms and similar devices. *Network* 1996; **16**.

42 Bounds, W. Female condoms. *Eur J Contracept Reprod Health Care* 1997; **2**: 113–16.

43 AIDSCAP. Women's Initiative. Female condom: from research to the marketplace. Chicago: Family Health International, 1997.

14 Can we tell them how to do it?

BRENDA SPENCER, JOHN GEROFI

Current quality standards for condoms require a very high level of compliance with "critical" tests. The international standard ISO 4074–1996[1] allows only 0.25 per cent to exhibit holes that can be found by filling the condom with water and rolling on absorbent paper. The standard also limits the proportion of condoms bursting at less than 16 litres (about 100 times the unstretched volume) under air inflation to 1 per cent. It is believed that these tests are a reliable indication of the condom's integrity, elasticity and strength.

Are instructions important?

Given the stringency of technical standards, many have concluded that reasons for condom failure must lie with the user. Indeed, research on the failure of condoms in preventing pregnancy has shown that the chief cause is non-use of the method. This is clear from the difference in pregnancy rates between consistent users and occasional users. For condoms as for all means of contraception, efficacy depends on the degree of motivation of the user.[2] As far as the prevention of sexually transmitted infections is concerned, the primary problem is once again non-use of the condom.[3] None the less, given the widespread recourse to use of the condom for HIV prevention, condom failure – that is breakage, slippage or spillage – has also become a major issue. A study conducted on a representative sample of the general population in France indicated that at last heterosexual intercourse 3.4 per cent of users experienced breakage and 1.1

per cent slippage.[4] Other recent prospective studies report even lower breakage,[5] while trials involving sex workers result in lower rates again.[6,7] From an epidemiological viewpoint, such low failure rates indicate excellent protection against many STIs (including HIV), but easier and more effective use and better products could further reduce risks and also the anxiety that individual users face on those rare occasions when the device fails.

The reasons for condom failure are hard to ascertain, given that numerous factors are no doubt at play, and that these factors are probably in large part "ergonomic", i.e. the result of the interaction between the characteristics of the product and the characteristics of the user.[8] In addition, it must be remembered that the objective of zero risk is unobtainable in any sphere of activity, and that a certain, if limited, level of failure is inevitable.

A recent study[9] seeking to identify users of condoms at risk of breakage or slippage hypothesised that the following practices were associated with condom failure:

* not opening the pack with fingers
* unrolling the condom before donning
* filling the condom with air or water
* donning condoms inside out
* using additional lubrication
* removing lubrication before or during use
* using condoms during particularly intense or lengthy coitus
* losing erection before withdrawal
* not holding the base of the condom during withdrawal
* re-using condoms.

In the study, increased failure rates were statistically associated with increased numbers of these selected practices. However, a direct link with any single practice was more difficult to establish. The methodological difficulties associated with this kind of study indicate that results should be interpreted with caution. For example, univariate analysis suggested that unrolling condoms before use was associated with breakage, but this was not supported on multivariate analysis. Moreover, in one of the countries where people were recruited for the study as many as 1 in 5 men reported unrolling before donning, but overall breakage rate in people from this country was lower than that of other countries studied where unrolling before use was less common.

Different studies tend to point to different factors related to condom failure, some related to practices and others to characteristics of the user, such as degree of experience of use, and education. A practice that is to be recommended in some circumstances, such as using additional lubricant for anal intercourse, may pose problems in others, such as vaginal intercourse with abundant natural lubrication.

Despite the complexity of the situation, and the lack of data indicating clear causality, the conclusion is often drawn that if people used condoms "correctly", the failure rates of condoms would be much lower than they currently are, and considerable zeal has therefore been applied to giving people "correct" instructions.

On the basis of which criteria might these "correct" instructions be determined? The content of condom instructions stems in the main from received wisdom, passed on from one set of writers to another. Instructions given by different suppliers and advisors differ, but there is sometimes a tendency to believe that more is better, and some sets of instructions appear to have been made by amalgamating all the others, past and present. Other sets appear to have been written by people who have never used a condom.

Results from a small body of research on the determinants of failure have become available in recent years. We may now compare these results with instructions generally given, but it should be pointed out that at their origin, the contents of instructions were essentially built up on "common sense" assumptions and not on scientific data. Consequently, some of the instructions to facilitate "correct" use have been irrelevant, and others potentially counter-productive. (One set included the directive to provide a towel previous to intercourse and carefully dry the penis after the event[10].)

For instructions to be effective, the content must be correct and understandable, as well as feasible and acceptable to the users. We should therefore ask:

- Are they read?
- Are they understood?
- Can and will they be put into practice? If so, have we correctly identified the techniques which will avoid breakage, slippage, and spillage?

Many standards dictate that instructions for use should always be supplied with condoms, yet overall it is probably fair to say, that if we know with certainty very little about what should absolutely be included in the instructions, we know even less about the "real-life" effectiveness of distributing written instructions in condom packs. The WHO Global Programme on AIDS commissioned research to determine how different presentations of instructions are perceived and made culturally acceptable.[11] Research on the readability of condom instructions to ascertain what level of education is required to follow them easily has also been conducted.[12,13] Yet overall, research on the effectiveness, perception, acceptability, and feasibility of condom instructions is rare.

Analysis of some typical instructions

Given the absence of clear data underlying condom instructions, it would seem a useful process to give more extensive thought to their face validity. We consider below one typical set of instructions widely used and accepted taken from a WHO publication on adapting instructions for different countries.[11] Each instruction (in italics) is considered individually and commented on.

Carefully open the package so condom does not tear   This instruction gives no information on HOW to avoid tearing the condom. It would be useful to say that the pack should be gripped by the sealed edge, outside the rolled condom. Depending on the type of pack used, one should recommend tearing along one edge, or tearing from the opening notch, where provided. This instruction destined to users raises the question of instructions destined to maufacturers, all of whom could make an effort to design their packaging in a more (hurried-)user-friendly way.

Nothing is included in these instructions about checking the direction of the unrolling before applying the condom and how this may be done. On removal from the sachet, the tip could be poking through the rolled condom the wrong way, usually rendering unrolling almost impossible. One commercial brand of condoms has the interesting instruction that if the condom does not unroll properly, then it is inside out, should be discarded and another one used. These product instructions are probably unusual in conceding that the condom could be the wrong way round, yet probability and the current methods of condom packaging dictate that 50 per cent of packs will be opened with the condom facing the wrong way up to unroll. (In 1999, a new package, from which the condom emerges right way up, was introduced by one manufacturer). It would therefore seem important to address this issue in the instructions.

Some instructions warn against use of scissors, teeth, etc. These implements should not be needed, but on the other hand, if the condom is moved away first, a scissor cut along one edge of the packet can be safe and effective.

Do not unroll condom before putting it on   Many instructions insist in this way that the condom must never be unrolled before being put on. This instruction is probably useful for most people, but there are exceptions. If a condom is being put on to a large glans, it is often helpful to unroll it partly and pull it over the glans, then unroll the rest. While most people unroll the condom onto the penis, others (generally sex workers putting condoms on clients) may successfully put on condoms by unrolling them first and putting them on like a sock.[14] The latter finding is in apparent contrast with the univariate analysis in the study described earlier.[9]

If not circumcised, pull foreskin back   Probably a useful suggestion, since it gives the penis the opportunity to move unrestricted. On the other hand, if the skin is pulled right back all the way to the base of the penis, then it will move forward again when it is released, and the rim of the condom could end up only 2 or 3 cm behind the glans, leaving most of the shaft exposed. The essence of the instruction should be to uncover the glans as far as practicable.

Squeeze tip of condom and put it on end of hard penis. Continue squeezing tip while unrolling condom until it covers all of penis   This instruction is mainly linked to the belief that if the tip is not squeezed, trapped air will increase the risk of breakage. Yet in the light of the substantial requirements of the inflation test indicated above, it is highly improbable that a few millilitres of air in the thickest part of the condom could cause breakage. Further, the air need not remain in the tip, it can distribute itself around the glans through the trough formed by the median raphe.

Even if the squeezing required above were necessary, it is implausible that it is necessary to hold the tip during unrolling. Once the air is out, and the condom is on the glans, the lubricant will hold it in place sufficiently to prevent the air rushing back and inflating the tip. Yet many instructions faithfully reproduce the injunction to keep squeezing the tip until the condom is unrolled to the base of the penis. This makes the process more complex, and in many cases, necessitates the use of three hands.

What, then, should be the process of unrolling? In general, we should recommend picking up the condom by the reservoir with the thumb and one finger of one hand, placing it on the glans, then beginning to unroll the condom with the other hand. At this point, it is then easier to continue unrolling using the thumb and one (or more) finger(s) of both hands until the condom is fully unrolled, or is within about 1 cm of the man's body. More experienced users may be able to use one hand, or form a ring with the thumb and forefinger to push the condom down. Skilled users may be able to perform the whole procedure of putting the condom on the glans and unrolling it with one hand.

Users should be aware of a particular problem which may be encountered during unrolling. If, during donning, the unrolled portion gets caught up by the fingers and pulled down over the part that is still rolled, further attempts to unroll the condom will result in the unrolled part being trapped between the roll and the penis. This effectively locks the condom and prevents further unrolling, unless it is re-rolled slightly.[15] It can be a relatively common occurrence, and condom users need to use an unrolling technique that avoids the fingers or hand sliding down the part that is already unrolled. Another cause of blockage during unrolling can be an adhesion between two layers of rubber in the roll, but this should occur rarely, if ever, in good quality products.

One set of complaints about faulty condoms was ascribed after investigation partly to instructions that said pull the condom down, rather than unroll.[15] The pulling action is likely to cause locking as above.

Anatomical factors that may cause some difficulties in application for a minority of users include:

• a very mobile foreskin
• an unusually large and tumescent glans
• a deep trough behind the corona of the glans
• a strongly tapered shaft.

Given the variations of anatomy, some individuals may find success using methods of condom application different from those above. Men finding that the condom is a little short, or that it tends to slip off, can unroll it fully, and then pull it down a little further by putting four fingers under the open end, and pulling.

Always put condom on before entering partner This is a compromise. For STI prevention, it is important to have the condom on before there is any contact between the penis and genital (or anal) areas. However, in contraceptive use, at least for those with good ejaculatory control, the condom may be put on later (see text below).

After ejaculating, hold rim of condom and pull penis out before penis gets soft. Slide condom off without spilling liquid (semen) inside Probably a good instruction. However, regarding spilling, apart from the aesthetics, the only really important thing is to avoid emptying the contents inside or close to the genitals or anus of the partner.

Throw away or bury the condom Pit latrines can also be used.

Do not use grease, oils, lotions, or petroleum jelly to make the condoms slippery: these make condoms break. Use only a jelly or cream that does not have oil in it Some users, especially anal users, find great benefit in the use of additional lubricants, and very often, common household materials like petroleum jelly or cooking oil have been used. It has been known for well over a decade that condoms were significantly weakened by contact with oils, especially light (low molecular weight) oils.

A recent study[16] of commonly found products that are likely to be used as condom lubricants showed that a very large percentage had a deleterious effect on the strength of condoms. Regrettably, there is no easy way that a consumer without some scientific knowledge can know whether a particular product is oil-based or not. Manufacturers could be more explicit in their labelling, and commercial outlets need to make an effort to associate the presentation of condoms with appropriate lubricants. Advice should also be given to avoid simultaneous use of any medications, pessaries, suppositories, etc. that may be oil-based. Water-based lubricants intended for sexual or medical use are too expensive for developing countries, and some advice on safe use of saliva would be desirable.

Studies have shown that for anal use, an appropriate lubricant reduces breakage and slippage.[17] In vaginal use, the situation is less clear as lubricant may increase the likelihood of slippage.[18,19] Clearly, it all depends on the abundance of natural lubrication. If intercourse is particularly prolonged, it is likely that the condom lubricant will dissipate, and there could be fatigue effects in the rubber. If the condom feels dry and uncomfortable, it should be replaced with a new one, or more lubricant added. Extraneous lubricant should be easily available, but it is inadvisable to recommend systematic use to all condom users, as has been put forward by some AIDS activist groups.

Use a condom each time you have sex   This is true for AIDS prevention, but not necessarily so for contraception (see text below).

Only use a condom once   This instruction is ambiguous as expressed here. The intent is to explain that a new condom should be used after each ejaculation.

Store condoms in a cool dry place   A good recommendation, but below about 25°C should be adequate.

Do not use condoms that may be old or damaged   Generally correct, but many an old condom would still be better than no condom at all. Use-by dates are not always based on firm data. Generally, good quality condoms will last five years in temperate climates, but their life in tropical countries may be less. Oxygen-impermeability of the pack contributes significantly to prolonging the shelf life.[20]

Do not use a condom if: the package is broken; the condom is brittle or dried out; the colour is uneven or changed; it is unusually sticky.
This instruction is more helpful than the previous one, since these are good warning signs of damaged condoms.

Additional points

In view of the apparent benefits of experience[14,21] and the differences among users, encouraging new users to practise first is important. This can be done alone, or, if desired, with a partner. Women can do it too, if there is a suitable penis model available. Such models need to have a realistic size, shape, and consistency.

If a particular condom is found uncomfortable, a different type may be tried. The width (circumference), shape, and the amount of lubricant are the most obvious properties that could affect comfort. Users should be aware that not all condoms are the same! Unfortunately, relatively little information is supplied by manufacturers in the packaging.

Contraception or prophylaxis: implications for condom instructions

Although the condom can play a dual role as a contraceptive and protection against STIs, people using the device solely for contraception can have more flexibility in their use than those wanting to protect against infection.

If there is any question of the need for prophylaxis, then a condom should be applied before any genital contact, and used on each occasion. However, for monogamous couples wishing solely to avoid conception, it is not necessary to have the condom on at first penetration, nor is it imperative to use a condom on each occasion of intercourse. This flexibility is never acknowledged in written instructions, and probably only extremely rarely in oral ones. None the less, many couples work it out for themselves, but optimal use of this combined approach depends on having a good understanding of the natural methods.

Given the importance of the AIDS pandemic, the urge on the part of professionals to err on the side of caution is understandable. Encouraging couples to develop an unchanging regime of condom use for maximum protection against all perils is, at first sight, the safest approach. It also provides prophylaxis without either party having to admit to, or accuse of, infidelity.

But the caution in this regard may also involve common (but probably mistaken) understandings regarding physiology, and also assumptions about the public's capacity to successfully take control of their own fertility.

Regarding the instruction of no genital contact prior to condom application, it is very widely believed that pre-ejaculatory fluid contains sperm capable of bringing about conception. Yet, as Potts and McDevitt[22] wrote in 1975, "the possibility of fertilising sperm being present in the pre-ejaculatory fluid has gained credence more by copying from textbook to textbook than by rational analysis". Major reviews have been unable to identify studies which substantiate this belief.[23] In one study with seropositive men, HIV was identified in pre-ejaculatory fluid in 50 per cent of the samples, and a few small clumps of sperm were said to have been found in 34 per cent of samples.[24] However, subsequent personal communication from the author of the study indicated that each sample contained fewer than 1000 spermatozoa, and in fact he suspected that the pre-ejaculatory sample had been contaminated by ejaculate. Moreover, the sperm seen would not be in sufficient quantity to cause conception. Compare the 1000 spermatozoa above with the 10 million spermatozoa per millilitre, below which infertility is usually diagnosed.

IPPF acknowledged in 1985 that the presence of sperm in pre-ejaculatory fluid "had not been well documented" but added that "a greater concern is that once penetration occurs the couple may not interrupt their activity to fit a condom". An allied concern is that "men differ in their ability to anticipate and control ejaculation".[23] On the other hand, in a recent Korean survey of health care workers, participants were given three choices for the best time to put on a condom. About 57 per cent chose before vaginal entry, 32 per cent said the mid-point of intercourse and 10 per cent said before ejaculation.[25]

The second debatable restriction on monogamous use is the requirement that a condom must be used on all occasions of intercourse. As sperm have limited life after ejaculation and a woman is only fertile on certain days, it is possible to identify days on which conception can occur, add a safety margin, and thus establish times when a condom is unnecessary. Newer techniques of fertility awareness to establish "safe" and "unsafe" periods, especially the sympto-thermal method, are considerably more reliable than the older calendar approaches.[26] Expertise in all these methods was originally located primarily in the Catholic community, which does not accept any method other than periodic abstinence. Some other family planning professionals may have been relatively slow to accept the efficacy of the newer natural methods. Thus users wishing to combine condoms with natural family planning may have had trouble finding good professional advice. Yet many couples who choose condoms for contraception do not use them on every occcasion of intercourse.[27–29,30] It is therefore constructive to show such couples how to minimise risk-taking, rather than simply labelling their behaviour irresponsible.

Should use of spermicides be recommended?

As both the condom and the spermicide were previously perceived as imperfect contraceptives, it was hypothesised that the use of both together would be considerably safer than either alone. The rationale is that if the condom leaks, breaks, or slips off, the spermicide will provide back-up protection. Simple probability calculations were done to illustrate that the two methods used together would give an efficacy similar to that of oral contraceptives. As a result many educators have recommended combined use of the two methods for maximum protection.[31]

Such calculations do not take into account the overall complexity of the situation. First, the most common reason for condom failure in use is likely to be non-use, rather than incorrect use or a faulty product. Furthermore, interruption of love-making is a common reason for disliking the condom, and spermicide application only adds further preparations and interruptions, thus reducing acceptability yet further, possibly resulting in decreased efficacy through decreased use. Second, the commonly used spermicides are surfactants, with irritant effects on mucous membrane (and skin). This may be compounded by mild abrasion from the condom. Side-effects for occasional users may be unnoticed, but for frequent users, such as sex workers, the spermicide may increase susceptibility to STIs. A recent study showed increased urinary tract infections among spermicide users.[32]

Applying additional spermicide can be avoided by using a spermicidally lubricated condom, but many manufacturers have trouble producing a uniform dispersion of spermicide in their lubricants. Others find it makes the individual foil packs deteriorate. Studies suggest that the quantity of spermicide applied to condoms by manufacturers is not sufficient to prevent STI transmission.[33,34]

It is not known whether a spermicide would work as a post-coital method to be used when and if a condom is found to have broken or slipped off.

What should be said?

Listed below is a useful basic set of instructions.

1 Open the pack by gripping it near the edge and tearing (at the notch/beside the seal, depending on the pack).
2 Check that the reservoir tip is poking out from the middle of the roll, to ensure that the condom can be unrolled.
3 Place the condom on the glans, and unroll on to the erect penis (before any genital contact fot STI prevention).

4 After ejaculation, and before the erection subsides, hold the rim of the condom on the penis and withdraw from your partner.

5 Dispose of the condom in a garbage receptacle (pit latrine).

Only the most important of the issues discussed previously should appear in the basic instructions on condom packaging and similar places. Other matters can be dealt with as answers to frequently asked questions, probably in separate documents, or orally by educators. Appropriate instructions for condom use should be succinct, since condoms are generally put on at a time when the users have other things on their minds, and do not want to spend time on elaborate procedures. Including additional steps which may theoretically improve effectiveness a little could complicate the instructions sufficiently to discourage people from following the instructions at all, or indeed from using condoms. Information that is relevant only to a small minority of users could have the same effect. As a final thought, it is reassuring to remember that most probably in condom use as in other areas of life "Practice makes perfect".

References

1 ISO 4074–1996 (several parts), *Rubber Condoms*, International Organisation for Standardisation, Geneva, 1996.

2 Jones E, Paul L, Westoff C. Contraceptive efficacy: the significance of method and motivation. *Stud Fam Plann* 1980; **11**: 39–50.

3 de Vincenci I. A longitudinal study of HIV transmission by heterosexual partners. *New Eng J Med* 1994; **331**(6): 341–6.

4 Messiah A, Dart T, Spencer BE, Warszawski J, and the French National Survey on Sexual Behaviour Group (ACSF). Condom breakage and slippage during heterosexual intercourse: a French National Survey. *Am J Public Health* 1997; **97**(3): 421–4.

5 Benton KWK, Joelley D, Smith AMA, Gerofi J, Moodie R. An actual use comparison of condoms meeting Australian and Swiss standards: results of a double-blind cross-over trial. *Int J STD AIDS* 1997; **8**: 427–31.

6 Albert AE, Warner DL, Hatcher RA, Trussell J, Bennett C. Condom use among female sex workers in Nevada's legal brothels *Am J Public Health* 1995; **85** (1 Nov.): 1514–20.

7 Richters J, Donovan B, Gerofi J, Watson L. Low condom breakage rate in commercial sex. *Lancet* 1988; 24 Dec: 1487–8.

8 Spencer B. The Condom Effectiveness Matrix: an analytical tool for defining condom research priorities. Paris: Les Editions INSERM, 1994, 83 pp.

9 Spuyt A, Steiner MJ, Joannis C, *et al*. Identifying condom users at risk for breakage and slippage: findings from three international sites. *Am J Public Health* 1998; **88**(2): 239–44.

10 Wright H. Barrier methods of contraception. *Br J Sex Med* 1981; **8**: 29–32.

11 Guide to Adapting Condom Instructions, WHO/GPA/CNP/92.1 World Health Organization, 1992.

12 Richwald GA, Walmsley MA, Coulson AH, Morisky DE. Are condom

instructions readable? Results of a readability survey. *Public Health Reports* 1988; **103**: 355–9.

13 Swanson JM, Forrest K, Ledbetter C, Hall S, Holstine EJ, Shafer MR. Readability of commercial and generic contraceptive instructions. *Image J Nurs Scholar* 1990; **22**(2): 96–100.

14 Richters J, Gerofi J, Donovan B. Why do condoms break or slip off in use? *Int J STD AIDS* 1995; **6**: 11–18.

15 Gerofi J, Deniaud F, Friel P. Interaction of condom design and user techniques and condom acceptability. *Contraception* 1995; **52**: 223–8.

16 Bernard P-F. Etude de l'influence des lubrifiants et médicaments à usage local, sur les caractéristiques physiques et mécaniques des préservatifs, Dossier 5120206, Document DMEE 12, Laboratoire National d'Essais, Paris, December 1997.

17 Dubois-Arber F, Jeannin A, Meystre-Agustoni G, *et al.* Evaluation of the AIDS prevention strategy in Switzerland, 5th assessment report 1993–95. Cah Rech Doc IUMSP no. 120b, 1997; 19–204.

18 Smith MA, Jolley D, Hocking J, Benton K, Gerofi J. Does additional lubricant affect condom slippage and breakage? *Int J STD AIDS* 1998; **9**: 330–5.

19 Spencer B. Doit-on conseiller l'utilisation de lubrifiant supplémentaire avec les préservatifs? *Transcriptase* 1994; **30**: 25–6.

20 Free MJ, Srisamang V, Vail J, Mercer D, Kotz R, Marlowe D. Latex rubber condoms: Predicting and extending shelf life. *Contraception* 1996; **53**: 221–9.

21 Lindberg LD, Sonnenstein FL, Ku L, Levine G. Young men's experience with condom breakage. *Fam Plann Perspect* 1997; **29**(3): 128–31.

22 Potts M, McDevitt J. A use-effectiveness trial of spermicidally lubricated condoms. *Contraception* 1975; **2**(6): 701–10.

23 Update on condoms – products, protection, promotion. Population Reports, Series H, No. 6, 10–5, September–October, 1982.

24 Pudney J, Oneta M, Mayer K, *et al.* Pre-ejaculatory fluid as potential vector for the sexual transmission of HIV-1. *Lancet* 1992; **340**, Dec: 1470.

25 Han JH, Park SH, Lee BS. Attitudes toward condom use of health centre workers in Korea. Institute of Reproductive Medicine and Population, Seoul National University, August 1998.

26 Population Reports. Periodic abstinence: how well do new approaches work? Population Information Program. The Johns Hopkins University, Baltimore. Series I, No. 3 September, 1981.

27 Coleman S. The cultural context of condom use in Japan. *Stud Fam Plann* 1981; **3**(1): 28–39.

28 Koyama I, Oato N. Condom use in Japan. In: Redford MH, Duncan GW, Prager DJ, eds. *The condom: increasing utilisation in the United States.* San Francisco Press Inc., 1974.

29 John A. Contraception in a practice community. *J Roy Coll Gen Pract* 1973; **23**: 665–79.

30 Peel J. The Hull Family Survey: II Family planning in the first five years of mariage. *J Biosoc Sci* 1972; **4**: 333–46.

31 Craig S, Hepburn S. The effectiveness of barrier methods of contraception with and without spermicide. *Contraception* 1982; **26**(4): 347–59.

32 Fihn SD, Boyko EJ, Normand EH, Yarbro P, Scholes D. Use of spermicide-coated condoms and other risk factors for urinary tract infection caused by *Staphylococcus saprophyticus, Arch Int Med* 1998; **158**(3): 281–7.

33 American Health Consultants. No added STD protection from spermicidal condoms. *Contracept Technol Update* 1998; **19**, 8 Aug: 105–6.

34 Trap R, Trap B, Petersen CS. The nonoxynol content in condoms is insufficient to inhibit HIV. *Ugeskrift for Laeger* 1990; **152**(46): 3464–6.

APPENDIX A

Table A.1 International and European condom standards compared[1,2]

Physical property		ISO 4074–1: 1996	EN 600: 1996
Dimensions:	Length	0–1/13 (AQL = 4.0%) <160 mm	Mean (N = 10) >170 mm
	Width	0–1/13 (AQL = 4.0%) outside nominal ±2 mm (25–35 mm from rim)	Mean (N = 10) within nominal ±2 mm (55–85 mm from rim)
Aqueous Leakage >25 mm from rim (or visible holes): 0–2/315 (AQL = 0.25%)		300 ml water hang/roll	300 ml water hang/roll; *or* 200 ml aqueous saline: if low electrical resistance then 300 ml hang/roll
Air Bursting (or leakage) <150 mm from closed end	Pressure	0–5/200 (AQL = 1.0%) <1.0 kPa	0–7/200 (AQL = 1.5%) <1.0 kPa
	Volume	0–5/200 (AQL = 1.0%) <16 litre (width = 52 mm)	and/or <18 litre
Oven-treated (70°C × 168 h)	Pressure	0–2/80 (AQL = 1.0%) <1.0 kPa	Not required
	Volume	0–2/80 (AQL = 1.0%) <16 litre (width = 52 mm)	
Tensile Breaking (20 mm long test-piece)	Elongation	Not required	Median (N = 13) >700 per cent
	Force		Median (N = 13) >39 newton (Strong >100 newton)
Oven-treated (70°C × 48 h)	Elongation	Not required	Median (N = 13) >700 per cent
	Force		Median (N = 13) >39 newton (Strong >100 newton)

APPENDIX B
Condom sampling, acceptable quality and limiting quality

ISO 4074 defines **Acceptable Quality Level** (AQL) thus: "When a continuous series of batches are considered, the quality level which, for the purposes of sampling inspection, is the limit of a satisfactory process average"[1]. More simply in practice, AQL means batch defectiveness (around 1.0 per cent) with a high chance of acceptance by a sampling plan.[3]

Producers seek to maximize the chance of accepting *good* batches (below AQL defectiveness), while consumers need to minimize the chance of accepting *bad* batches (defectiveness over four times AQL). The *producer's* risk is 95 per cent acceptable batch defectiveness (AQ 95); the *consumer's* risk is 5 per cent acceptable batch defectiveness (**Limiting Quality**, LQ 5).

For air-tested condom *weakness* (AQL = 1.0 per cent), ISO 4074 prescribes sampling at General Inspection Level I (sample density). From a typical batch (1 000 gross = 144 000 condoms), that means randomly sampling 200 specimens, and permitting 0–5 air-tested defectives. This Single Sampling plan accepts over 98 per cent of 1.0 per cent defective batches; 95 per cent of 1.3 per cent defective batches; and 5 per cent of 5.2 per cent defective batches (LQ 5 = 5.2 times AQL).

For an AQL of 1.0 per cent, Table B.1 shows 1.0 per cent defective batch acceptability increasing with sample size, from 88 per cent for none out of 13 defective, to 99 per cent for 0–10 defectives out of 500 condoms tested, while consumer protection increases (LQ 5 decreasing, from over 20 times AQL, to 3 times AQL).

For condom *length* under 160 mm, and specimens over 2 mm outside nominal *width* (AQL = 4.0 per cent), ISO 4074 prescribes a low inspection level, permitting 0–1 out of 13 defective (AQ 95 = 2.8 per cent; but LQ 5 = 32 per cent = 8 times AQL). For water-tested condom *leakage* (AQL = 0.25 per cent), ISO 4074 and EN 600 typically permit 0–2 out of 315 defectives (AQ 95 = 0.26 per cent; but LQ 5 = 2.0 per cent = 8 times AQL).

For *visibly defective* condoms, EN ISO 4074 may prescribe an AQL of 1.0 per cent, allowing 7 defectives out of 315 test specimens (LQ 5 = 4.1 times AQL).

221

Table B.1   Condom Single Sampling plans for Normal inspection at General Inspection Level I (AQL = 1.0 per cent)

Batch size (Number of Condoms)	Sample size (Number of test-condoms)		1.0 per cent defective batch **Acceptability** (per cent)	Batch acceptability: **Defectiveness** (per cent)	
	Total	Defective (maximum)		95 per cent (AQ 95):	5 per cent (LQ 5):
500 or less	13	0	87.8	0.4	20.6
501–3 200	50	1	91.1	0.7	9.1
3 201–10 000	80	2	95.3	1.0	7.7
10 001–35 000	125	3	96.3	1.1	6.1
35 001–150 000[a]	200	5	98.4	1.3	5.2
150 001–500 000	315	7	98.5	1.3	4.1
500 001 or more	500	10	98.7	1.2	3.4

[a] Typical condom batch size.

For sample-testing consecutive batches, EN ISO 4074 may prescribe tighter Switching Rules.[3] For checking *isolated* batches, a higher sample density (General Inspection Level II) is preferable: with an AQL of 1.0 per cent typically permitting 10 out of 500 defectives (LQ 5 = 3.4 times AQL).

Appendix References

1 International Organization for Standardization. International Standard ISO 4074–1: 1996 *Rubber condoms – Part 1: Requirements*. Geneva: ISO, 1996.
2 Comité Européen de Normalisation. European Standard EN 600: 1996 *Natural rubber latex male condoms*. Brussels: CEN, 1996.
3 International Organization for Standardization. International Standard ISO 2859–1: 1989 *Sampling procedures for inspection by attributes – Part 1: Sampling plans indexed by acceptable quality level (AQL) for lot-by-lot inspection*. Geneva: ISO, 1989.

Index